	WOOD	FIRE	EART	METAL	WAT	TON CAT	SEDAT	SOUR	ASS	A	LUO	HUN	ENT	EXIT	LO MEL	UP ME P
Lung	L11	L10	L9	L8	L5	L9	L5	L9	B13	L1	L7	L6	L1	L7	...	...
Spleen	Sp1	Sp2	Sp3	Sp5	Sp9	Sp2	Sp5	Sp3	B20	Liv13	Sp4	Sp8	Sp1	Sp21	...	...
Heart	H9	H8	H7	H4	H3	H9	H7	H7	B15	Cv14	H5	H6	H1	H9	...	...
Kidney	K1	K2	K6	K7	K10	K7	K1	K6	B23	G25	K5	K1	K1	K22	...	...
Pericardium	P9	P8	P7	P5	P3	P9	P7	P7	B14	Cv17	P6	P4	P1	P8	...	...
Liver	Liv1	Liv2	Liv3	Liv4	Liv8	Liv8	Liv2	Liv3	B18	Liv14	Liv5	Liv6	Liv1	Liv14	...	...
	METAL	WATER	WOOD	FIRE	EARTH											
Large intestine	Li1	Li2	Li3	Li5	Li11	Li11	Li2	Li4	B25	S25	Li6	Li7	Li4	Li20	S37	Li11
Stomach	S45	S44	S43	S41	S36	S41	S45	S42	B21	Cv12	S40	S34	S1	S42	S36	
Small intestine	Si1	Si2	Si3	Si5	Si8	Si3	Si8	Si4	B27	Cv4	Si7	Si6	Si1	Si19	S39	Si8
Bladder	B67	B66	B65	B60	B54	B67	B65	B64	B28	Cv3	B58	B63	B1	B67	B54	
Triple warmer	T1	T2	T3	T6	T10	T3	T10	T4	B22	Cv5	T5	T7	T1	T23	B53	T10
Gall bladder	G44	G43	G41	G38	G34	G43	G38	G40	B19	G24	G37	G36	G1	G41	G34	

Acupuncture Therapy

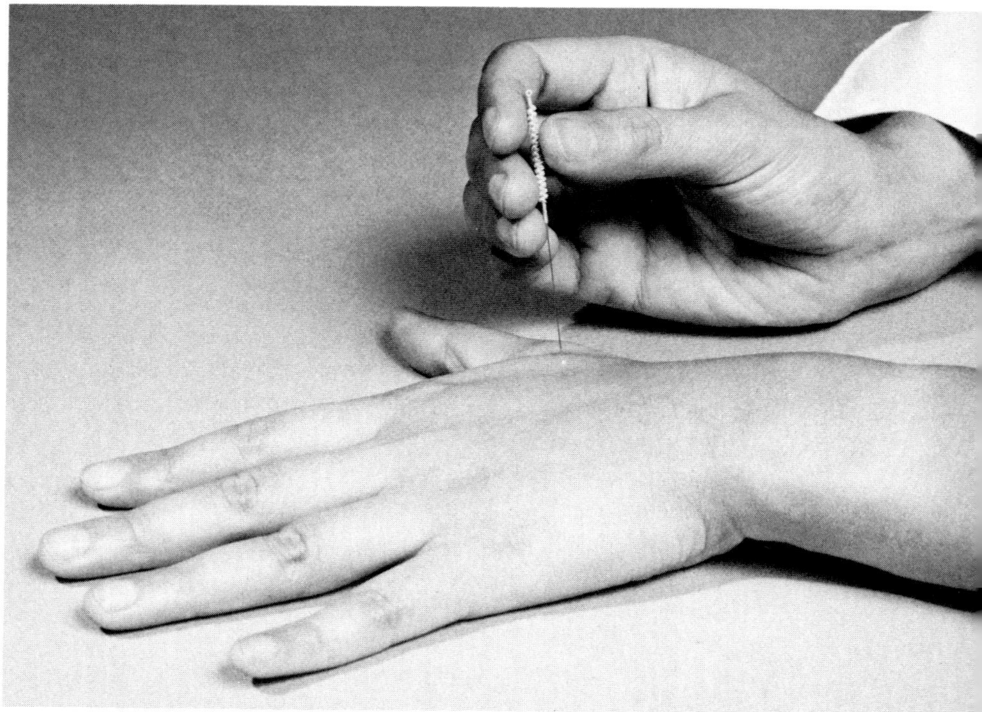

Temple University Press *Philadelphia*

Acupuncture Therapy

Current Chinese Practice

Second Edition,
Revised and Enlarged

Leong T. Tan
Margaret Y.-C. Tan
Ilza Veith

Foreword by Walter R. Tkach, M.D.

Temple University Press, Philadelphia 19122

Published 1973. Fourth impression 1975. Second edition 1976
Printed in the United States of America

International Standard Book Number: 0–87722–064–6
Library of Congress Catalog Card Number: 75–30280

LEONG T. TAN, M.D., F.A.C.S., is a urologist practicing in San Francisco. MARGARET Y.-C. TAN, M.S., is an acupuncturist in the Acupuncture Research Clinic at the University of California San Francisco. ILZA VEITH, M.A., Ph.D., D. Med. Sc., is professor and vice chairman of the Department of the History of Health Sciences at the University of California San Francisco and a leading authority on oriental medicine. She has written many books and articles and is the translator of *The Yellow Emperor's Classic of Internal Medicine*.

Again

TO HANS

A Man for All Seasons

CONTENTS

Foreword *ix*
Preface to the Second Edition *xi*
Preface to the First Edition *xv*
Introduction *3*
1 The Essentials of Acupuncture *21*
Acupuncture Needles *21*
Techniques of Acupuncture *22*
Moxibustion *26*
Electric Acupuncture *26*
Possible Complications of Acupuncture *27*
Identification of Acupuncture Points *28*
2 Most Commonly Used Acupuncture Points *33*
Points of the Head and Neck *33*
Points of the Upper Extremity *48*
Points of the Lower Extremity *70*
Points of the Chest and Abdomen *95*
Points of the Back *101*
Points of the External Ear *112*
3 Less Commonly Used Acupuncture Points *121*
4 Diseases and Symptoms Amenable to Acupuncture Therapy *199*
Selection of Acupuncture Points for Treatment *199*
List of Diseases and Symptoms *203*

5 Acupuncture-Anesthesia *221*
Principles of Acupuncture-Anesthesia *222*
Selection of Acupuncture Points *223*
Current Chinese Observations on the Mechanism(s) of Acupuncture-Analgesia *234*

Bibliography *241*
Index of Most Commonly Used Acupuncture Points *249*
Index of Diseases and Symptoms *257*

FOREWORD

The recent resurgence of interest in acupuncture therapy may very well be due to President Richard Nixon's journey to the People's Republic of China. It has also been due to articles published by Dr. E. Grey Dimond and Dr. Paul Dudley White. The most scholarly presentation was made by Dr. Dimond in his articles in the *Journal of the American Medical Association.*

After we had visited the Friendship Hospital in Peking, I immediately reported to the President and related to him the operative procedures that we had observed. He was intensely interested, and the request was made that I review my notes and write a summary that would be of interest in America. This was done in articles in *Today's Health* and another widely disseminated journal. The happy surprise was the great number of physicians as well as members of the general public who wrote and asked for more information and about the possibility of visiting China to study the acupuncture procedure as it was used in anesthesia and for the relief of pain. Literally thousands of letters were received.

Three surgical procedures were observed, and when the value of the new anesthetic technique was realized, it was obvious that the medical profession outside of China could very well utilize this method. It is not a perfect anesthetic procedure, but the benefits derived from it were certainly impressive. As I thought about acupuncture-anesthesia in the months following, I realized that this was not anesthesia in the sense that we would describe it. I suggested to Dr. Ilza Veith that a new word should be coined. She suggested acupuncture-analgesia, but as we come to know more about it, I would hope that a more fitting and descriptive term will be found.

In the eight days that we spent in the People's Republic of China this new modality was discussed many times with the Chinese physicians. It was obvious that it had its finest application in the relief of pain. They made no extravagant claims as to cures for cancer, heart disease, and other illnesses that befall mankind. It appeared that they knew exactly at that time what they had and what they could do with it. It is my hope that in the near future we will be able to send a team to the People's Republic of China to study this procedure in detail in order to become proficient and to teach American physicians the value of acupuncture therapy and particularly its application to anesthesia.

Doctors Leong T. Tan and Ilza Veith and Mrs. Margaret Y.-C. Tan have written an excellent text and assembled what is probably our total knowledge of acupuncture outside of the People's Republic of China.

WALTER R. TKACH, M.D.

The White House
Spring, 1973

PREFACE TO THE SECOND EDITION

Aspirin is not a cure-all! Nor is acupuncture! Any different approach is misguided, possibly even of questionable ethics. The truly immense attention, almost excitement, of the public regarding this therapy, which was previously little known in America, has produced a rather hectic response from certain sectors of the healing profession. Such response would seem to be somewhat inappropriate for various reasons: the first being that the overwhelming majority of physicians and dentists in this country has no well-founded knowledge of, or experience with, acupuncture; the second being that most facilities currently available for study and instruction in this art must by all professional standards appear insufficient and underdeveloped, to say the least.

The wish to help narrow the gap between the clamor for treatment and the dearth of competent practitioners induced the authors of *Acupuncture Therapy: Current Chinese Practice* to write this description of an ongoing therapeutic method which, for all intents and purposes, has been successfully employed from before the dawn of Chinese history to the present day.

The eager response to the first edition of the book, which necessitated several subsequent printings, has provided the encouragement for the preparation of this extended and revised edition. In taking cognizance of certain questions raised by interested reviewers, the authors wish to state again that this book deals with acupuncture as it is now performed and applied within the framework of the medical system of the People's Republic of China. With the sometimes heated debate in progress about the pros and cons of the method, the authors deem it untimely to editorialize on the contents of their Chinese sources. The book, including this new edition, remains therefore wholly informative.

So far as new material is concerned, an entirely new chapter, in which all of the remaining known acupuncture points of the body are compiled, forms part of the new edition. Although these points are less frequently used, the practitioner may find it of interest and value to possess this additional information.

In the "Index of Most Commonly Used Acupuncture Points," the authors decided to add to the anatomical numbers a listing of the so-called Meridian numbers for comparison. This system of numbering acupuncture points was first introduced by nineteenth-century French investigators for readers unfamiliar with the Chinese language and is frequently found in modern European literature. Even if some students of acupuncture find it easier to memorize numbered points such as "Gallbladder 5" or "Large Intestine 4," it should be borne in mind that a logical connection between such organs and the functions the points are to perform does not necessarily exist. This numbering system is entirely for the convenience of Western students of acupuncture.

In the field of acupuncture-analgesia (anesthesia) for surgical intervention additional material has become available from China, since the book was first published. In view of the fact that analgesia-inducing acupuncture has in the meantime been admitted and successfully applied in numerous clinics, university and other hospitals, here and abroad, especially in cardio-vascular and thoracic surgery performed in Germany, the authors are particularly gratified at being in a position to present this important addition for the benefit of all concerned.

The extension also had to consider developments in the legal field with regard to the practice of acupuncture. Since the day when California was the first state to pass laws on this subject, practically every state in the Union, as well as the federal government, has taken regulatory action in one form or another. It would seem, though, that at present, the matter is still in a state of flux with more legislative attention to be expected.

An examination of contemporary acupuncture in this country appears to show that the public demand for access to this therapy has gone far beyond the services the medical profession is able to provide. Obviously the cause for this situation is the inadequate number of competent acupuncturists authorized to practice, and it is the want of training facilities which lies at the root of the problem. Yet the principal purveyor of medical education (i.e., academic medicine) so far has reacted mainly by getting involved in theoretical investigations into the physiological and neurological aspects of this field. In pursuing the engrossing question, Why does acupuncture work? little or nothing has transpired that would point to a concern for How is it performed? To all appearances, little has yet been undertaken towards setting up academically acceptable facilities for systematic instruction in, and study of, the practice of this time-honored therapeutic modality.

Leong T. Tan, M.D. F.A.C.S.
Margaret Y.-C. Tan, M.S.
Ilza Veith, M.A., PH.D., D. MED. SC.

San Francisco
Spring, 1976

PREFACE TO THE FIRST EDITION

Until recently, a monograph on acupuncture would have attracted little or no interest in the Western world, much less in the United States. Acupuncture, it appeared, was a phenomenon that belonged to the realm of folklore, fantasy, mysticism, and indeed, even witchcraft. "A lot of hocus pocus" seemed to be the prevailing comment. In reality, however, acupuncture is a traditional mode of medical treatment in China, the practice of which has existed for thousands of years. Millions of patients, from personal experiences, can attest to the effect of needles, properly inserted at specific locations of the body: the palliation of certain afflictions, the alleviation of pain, and in recent years, the medical wonder of acupuncture-anesthesia or acupuncture-analgesia. As a simple, efficient, and, more important, effective means of medical therapy, acupuncture has successfully withstood the test of time, of scrutiny, and of acceptance. To those who remain skeptical of, or are baffled by, its accomplishments, this ancient art of healing deserves serious, responsible, and objective evaluation of its merits.

Many books have been written on this subject, both in Oriental and in Western languages. Judging from comments made by prospective students of this mode of therapy as well as from personal investigation of available literature, the authors found wanting an adequate source of instruction on the practical aspects of acupuncture treatment in the Western texts, specifically in the English language. It was to fill this particular void that the authors embarked on the preparation of this book. To this end, several current Chinese texts on acupuncture have been reviewed in detail and selectively translated. Information so gained forms the contents of this book.

As a medical procedure, the insertion and manipulation of acupuncture needles is fairly simple. For all practical purposes, no hazard to the general health of the patient is incurred provided, of course, that acupuncture is correctly practiced. On the strength of its simplicity and effectiveness, acupuncture has enjoyed a wide acceptance as a home cure performed by self-taught friends and family members. The problem that arises, however, is that acupuncture is by no means a cure-all. Serious pathological conditions that will not yield to needle treatment may be overlooked and remain undiagnosed by a medically untrained operator. A professional diagnosis is therefore at least as important for acupuncture therapy as it is for any other kind of medical intervention.

The present reception of acupuncture in Western, especially in American, scientific society raises memories of previous medical innovations, such as vaccination, anesthesia, antisepsis, chemotherapy, insulin, and antibiotics, to name just a few. Opinion of these innovations often gyrated between "myth" and "miracle." All were hotly debated, but it was a prominent American surgeon, John Collins Warren, who exclaimed after his first operation with ether anesthesia in 1846: "Gentlemen, this is no humbug!" Time will tell whether or not acupuncture will enter our vocabulary of medical household words and be taken for granted as a therapeutic method along with so many others.

Leong T. Tan, M.D., F.A.C.S.
Margaret Y.-C. Tan, M.S.
Ilza Veith, M.A., PH.D., D. MED. SC.

San Francisco
Summer, 1973

Acupuncture Therapy

INTRODUCTION

AMERICAN "DISCOVERY" OF ACUPUNCTURE

No aspect of the American rapprochement with China, including President Nixon's historic visit in February 1972, has caught the interest of the American public as much as have news items—quite incidental indeed—about the medical experience of a distinguished American correspondent. By suffering an appendicitis and undergoing an appendectomy, James Reston of the *New York Times* "discovered" acupuncture, a "discovery" that was made anew by most subsequent American visitors to China in 1971–72, including President Nixon.

In fact, some of those who discovered acupuncture in the year of rapprochement were not completely incorrect in regarding it as a new modality that was somehow associated with Chairman Mao. But only acupuncture-anesthesia is actually a new phenomenon, hardly more than ten years old, and almost unknown outside of China proper. This aspect of acupuncture, important as it is, is really an innovation upon an ancient method of treatment, for acupuncture as an analgesic and as therapy stems from the neolithic age and is therefore at least seven thousand years old. Proof for this surprising statement is the existence of acupuncture needles made of flint, bone, and slivers of bamboo, long before the discovery of metal.

It is interesting that of all Western nations, scarcely any but the United States would have reacted to the sight of acupuncture with as much amazement and surprise. In most countries of Europe, especially France, Germany, Austria, England, and Russia, acupuncture therapy has long been known and practiced by physicians without discrimination from their scientific medical colleagues. Except for Russia, which adopted acupuncture as late as 1959, the other European countries became acquainted with this Chinese practice in the seventeenth and eighteenth centuries, when their colonial, diplomatic, or religious representatives returned from the Far East and spoke highly of the therapeutic methods they had observed. Here it should be stressed that the original oriental application of acupuncture was for the alleviation of the pains of arthritis, gout, and gastro-intestinal disturbances.

It was probably just because of these specific applications that acupuncture found such an interested reception in Europe, for gout in particular was a major bane of the well-born, of scholars, and especially of the most prominent of the physicians. As medical records and statistics had not come into use in those centuries, we do not know how effective acupuncture was in actually bringing relief from these painful afflictions, nor do we have these answers today.

WHAT IS ACUPUNCTURE?

Before continuing the story of acupuncture in the West, a few words should be said about the actual value of, and the rationale for, this procedure.

As we said above, acupuncture is part of the ancient Chinese medical system reaching back into prehistoric times. Its earliest documentation may be found in a medical treatise which was written in the third or fourth century B.C., *The Yellow Emperor's Classic of Internal Medicine.* According to Webster, the word "acupuncture" is derived from the Latin word *acus,* the needle, and *punctura,* a pricking, and means "a puncturing of bodily tissue for the relief of pain." It is performed by inserting sharp needles of various lengths into one or several of hundreds of points located all over the body, including the head and the extremities. These needles are inserted to various depths, rotated, left in situ, or immediately withdrawn.

It is difficult to find the rationale for the introduction of this uncommon therapy. Even in *The Yellow Emperor's Classic of Internal Medicine,* no such explanation is given. At the time this work was written, acupuncture must have been such a well-known form of therapy that explanations of its origin were considered unnecessary. In the course of history, however, a number of legends have arisen which furnish spurious (or perhaps even valid) explanations. The one most frequently cited is that ancient Chinese warriors, after having been injured by arrows in a variety of places, noticed the disappearance of pains of long standing and hence figured out a cause-and-effect relationship between the arrow wound and the unexpected amelioration or cure of their pains. Rather than believing in events that can scarcely be documented, it seems wiser to search for a rationale in the medical philosophy of the ancient Far East. Thus, what seems more likely than the apocryphal warriors is the early observation of the analgesic effect of massage, which also originated in China, that is, the kneading of specific parts of the body to bring about general relaxation and alleviation of pain.

As long as we do not have a documented Chinese history of the discovery of acupuncture, it will be important to understand its application and curative effect in terms of the ancient oriental natural philosophy. It needs to be stressed that the rationale for acupuncture is totally unrelated to any Western reasons for inserting needles into the human body: acupuncture needles are not hollow and do not serve to convey any material into the body, nor are they used to withdraw any body fluid. Attempts to bring acupuncture within the framework of modern medical science have as yet not solved the enigma.

All traditional Chinese medicine is based on the concept that, in composition and function, man is a microcosmic image of the universe and subject to identical laws. From time immemorial the Chinese were awed by the immutable course of nature, which they thought to be guided by *Tao* 道, the Way. Tao prevailed in the creation of the world out of a state of chaos; Tao causes the ever-recurring changes from day to night, from light to darkness, from life to death, and is present in the coexistence of good and evil, of male and female. The two forces through which Tao acts were named *Yin* 陰 and *Yang* 陽; Yin, the female element, possesses all the negative qualities, and Yang, the male element, all the positive qualities. Since Tao was thought to be a unitary principle, neither of its two components ever existed alone, and in an absolute state. Even in the male there was an admixture of the female element; and in the female an admixture of the male.

In the universe, the harmonious working of the dual forces Yin and Yang expressed itself in the waning and waxing of the moon, the rising and setting of the sun, the growing and ripening of the crops and countless other sequential natural phenomena. Droughts, floods, storms, tidal waves, earthquakes and other disasters of nature were thought to be the result of an imbalance of Yin and Yang. Similarly, in man and beast, health resulted from the balance of the Yin and the Yang, and all diseases were thought to be due to a dyscrasia of these forces.

In the physical body, both human and animal, this need for homeostasis as a prerequisite for health is expressed also in the concept of the vital essence *ch'i* 氣, consisting of a harmonious mixture of Yin and Yang, which was believed to be conveyed through twelve pairs of main ducts, plus two trunk ducts, which run in the front and back midline of the body. In the Western world these ducts or channels have come to be designated as "meridians." The meridians emerge at the surface of the body at a certain number of carefully designated and presumably sensitive places which subsequently became known as acupuncture points. These traditionally numbered 365, to correspond with the number of days in the solar year.

As a consequence of the belief of disease being due to dyscrasia, the Chinese did not recognize a variety of diseases. They saw only disease as such, brought about by one cause—the disequilibrium of Yin and Yang within the vital force—which could affect different parts of the body. A similar relationship was thought to exist between the pulse and each of the internal organs. Each wrist was assumed to contain not one but six pulses and both wrists, that is, twelve pulses, had to be palpated by the physician. Since the twelve pairs of meridians conveying the Yin and Yang were held to have a direct connection with every organ and part of the body, it was logical to assume that these channels furnished the easiest access to the seat of the disturbance. In response to individual symptoms, specific points were chosen for each needling treatment. By inserting needles into one or several points and by leaving them in situ for a certain length of time, the equilibrium of Yin and Yang was expected to be restored, possibly by the escape of disharmonious combinations.

It needs further to be pointed out, as we gratefully acknowledge Dr. Joseph Needham's personal communication, that the selection of acupuncture points must be based on correct diagnosis, which was not only founded on the very characteristic sphygmology, but also on the apparent interaction among the various organ systems that were distinguished in the traditional Chinese anatomy. These organ systems, the five *tsang* (脏) or main organs, were held to consist of the heart, the liver, the spleen, the lungs and the kidneys. All of these were thought to belong to the realm of Yin and were credited with the capacity of storing but not of elimination. In addition, there are six other internal organ systems, known as *fu* (腑) which comprise the gall bladder, the urinary bladder, the stomach, the large intestine, the small intestine, and the mysterious organ, known as the "three burning spaces" (三焦), the "three foci," or the "triple warmer." The six fu organs belong to Yin and have the capacity to eliminate but not to store.

Beyond the interaction of the five tsang and the six fu, the ancient Chinese had fairly precise ideas about the movement of ch'i, the spirit or energy of life, and the *hsüeh,* blood. It seems that from several centuries before our era onwards this movement was visualized as a circulation taking place at a rate of about sixty times slower than the circulation discovered by William Harvey.

The network of channels distributing the vital essence ch'i throughout the body interconnects with the vascular and neurological system. Furthermore, the network is subject to seasonal lunar, annual, and circadian cycles.

It is extremely difficult to express the concepts of these traditional temporal circulations in adequate Western terminology, unless we realize that they were precognitions of what we now know as circadian clocks and monthly endocrine rhythms.

Each of these points was believed to be the direct exponent of a specific and possibly diseased organ within the body. Such a belief appears to demonstrate a complete and deliberate disregard for any knowledge of the structure and function of the human body, in favor of a theory which obviated a systematic study of anatomy. This disregard persisted because anatomical dissection was taboo among the ancient Chinese, whose veneration of the ancestral personality demanded the burial of an inviolate body, that is, a body untouched by the probing instruments of anatomical dissection, or even the knife of the surgeon. It was thus possible to assume the actual existence of twelve pairs of meridians as channels for the vital essence which transported the life force of man.

Belief in the existence of the meridians persisted even after the introduction of the study of anatomy and scientific medicine into China, and after it had become evident that the meridians and acupuncture points could not actually be demonstrated as discrete anatomical structures. Only very recently a Korean researcher, Kim Bong-han, claimed to have discovered and demonstrated the existence of additional meridians along which he traced what he called the "Bong-han" points.

SCIENTIFIC THEORIES ON ACUPUNCTURE

Western medicine cannot help but speculate about the scientific secret of acupuncture, and several theories have been suggested to account for the uncanny success of the oriental procedure.

Lacking a knowledge of the nature and function of the central nervous system and of the brain, which was not considered one of the major organs of the body, the traditional Chinese practitioners of acupuncture had to work with the concepts inherent in their philosophical theories of man's bodily function. Divested from concepts of Yin and Yang and "vital essence," however, the idea of dermal representation of internal organs in the cerebral cortex is not as fanciful as it appears at first glance. The work of men of such scientific sophistication as Rasmussen and Penfield showed twenty-five years ago that each area of the surface of the skin is represented by a corresponding area in the cerebral cortex. This correspondence between skin and cerebral cortex probably also accounts for the beneficial effect of massage.

While the Rasmussen-Penfield theory was not specifically intended to explain acupuncture but may well be applied to it, other investigators have concentrated upon finding a physiological explanation for acupuncture-analgesia.

As was to be expected, the arrival of modern Western scientific medicine in China reduced the importance of the disequilibrium of Yin and Yang as pathogenic factors and made it desirable to look for scientific reasons for the efficacy of acupuncture treatment. This is all the more the case since acupuncture has reached the Western world, and especially the United States. Most frequently quoted among these scientific reasons is the hypothesis of R. Melzack of McGill University and Patrick Wall of the University College in London, whose studies on the physiology of pain yielded the gate control theory. The so-called Melzack-Wall theory suggests that the pathway of pain to the brain is determined by a "gate control cell" in the substantia gelatinosa in the dorsal horn of the spinal cord.

Although a certain element of scientific speculation remains in this proposition, a connection with acupuncture was developed on the basis of the Melzack-Wall theory. According to reports of recent visitors to the People's Republic of China, Chinese investigators have been proceeding along this line of thought in considering the role of cortex, thalamus and hypothalamus. In the United States, two scientists in Michigan, Dr. Calvin H. Chen, a professor at Wayne State University and assistant medical superintendent at Northville State Hospital, and Dr. Pang L. Man of the same institution, have formulated a concept to establish the thalamus as a second gate and have hence termed their hypothesis the "two-gate control theory."

It is important also to note here that according to the latter theory acupuncture needles produce only a mild, fairly painless stimulation causing the gates to be closed, so that painful sensations cannot pass through.

Further speculations on this theory have appeared in an article by H. C. Tien. Important research is also being conducted under the auspices of the National Institutes of Health.

In all probability none of the above mentioned theories on the neurophysiological mechanism of acupuncture is the last word in the explanation of the needle therapy, and it is entirely uncertain whether it will eventually be one or several investigators in the People's Republic of China or Western researchers who will succeed in finding the scientific basis for this mysterious operation. The immediate and perhaps somewhat simplistic response of many American physicians who are not themselves familiar with acupuncture has often been that it can simply be equated with hypnosis, i.e., suggestion. This "explanation" can hardly be considered the correct one, since acupuncture is effective in the treatment of infants and also of a great variety of animals. Neither infants nor animals have as yet been known to be susceptible to hypnosis. In fact, Tibetan and Mongolian nomads have for centuries succeeded in producing insensibility to pain in their horses for purposes of veterinary intervention with acupuncture.

Moreover, in modern pain research, the difference between psychogenic pain and somatogenic pain is considered to be increasingly less significant. It is difficult, if not impossible, to dissociate the mind from painful ailments. As far as psychosomatic aspects of acupuncture therapy are concerned, it stands to reason that Mao Tse-tung's personal interest in the resurgence and extension of acupuncture endows the Chinese patient with such complete confidence in the procedure that he is free even of pre-operative apprehension. So far as the treatment of emotional illness is concerned, acupuncture seems to be effective in the relief of a great many psychogenic dysfunctions, such as frigidity and impotence, obesity and anorexia nervosa, insomnia and excessive fatigue, asthma, and migraine.

Acupuncture research is also going forward in all the European countries where it has been practiced so far. It is interesting to note that precisely those European nations which represent the cradle of modern medical science have accepted acupuncture as one of the therapeutic modalities open to the medical profession. The same is true in Japan, where acupuncturist physicians practice side by side with their Western-trained colleagues. This is because, centuries ago, Chinese medicine, and with it acupuncture, has found its way into all Asian countries which were pervaded by Chinese culture: Korea, Taiwan—in fact, all of Southeast Asia—but chiefly Japan. The most important researches, as has to be expected, are being conducted in the People's Republic of China; these findings are summarized in the chapter dealing with acupuncture-anesthesia.

MOXIBUSTION

Moxibustion is another form of therapy which developed in China in conjunction with acupuncture. It is the application to the established acupuncture points of small combustible cones of dried leaves of *Artemisia vulgaris,* or wormwood, which are ignited and burned down to the skin until a blister forms. Like acupuncture, moxibustion is also intended to restore homeostasis to the body. It was enthusiastically received in Japan, where it has continued to be practiced in its original form as an alternative to acupuncture, regardless of the burn scars that result. (The word "moxa" is derived from the Japanese *mogusa* "burning herb.") In China, on the other hand, moxibustion has continued in a somewhat attenuated form. Instead of bringing the burning moxa stick so close to the skin that a blister results, the smoldering moxa has been removed from the skin and is now used almost exclusively for heating the needles or warming the acupuncture point from a distance.

PRACTICAL APPLICATION

The sudden flurry of interest in the United States in the practice of acupuncture has caused many desperately ill patients to seek this apparent cure-all. In this they were disappointed, as there are very few physicians in the United States who are skilled acupuncturists. With the increasing demand for this method of treatment, however, many American physicians have evinced an interest in the actual techniques of acupuncture, which have so far been the domain of anonymous practitioners within the Chinese communities in this country. The few licensed physicians skilled in acupuncture usually have had full-time obligations in other fields of medicine, and practiced acupuncture as a "side-line" only. The many textbooks on acupuncture which have been published in France, Germany, Japan, and China are generally inaccessible to American readers. But quite apart from the linguistic or cultural differences that separate the American reader from the European and Oriental publications, it should be stressed that these are largely based upon the ancient traditional methods of acupuncture. In the People's Republic of China acupuncture therapy has undergone considerable refinement. From among the many hundreds of traditional acupuncture points those have been chosen which have come to be known as most effective in pain therapy and anesthesia. In addition to narrowing down and refining the number of ancient points, the Chinese have added new points which are not hallowed by tradition but which have yielded unexpectedly favorable results.

A number of these points also come into play in acupuncture anesthesia, and it is this facet of acupuncture that has most deeply impressed Western medical observers on their visits to the People's

Republic of China. Strictly speaking, the expression "acupuncture-anesthesia," though widely used, is somewhat of a misnomer. The proper nomenclature should probably be acupuncture-analgesia. Since no paralysis of the nerve centers with consequent muscle relaxation, loss of consciousness and of all sensations occurs as it does in inhalation anesthesia, the patient remains fully conscious and aware that he is being operated upon. However, he does not feel the pain or discomfort that would ordinarily be felt in surgery. Acupuncture preparatory to and during the operation results in analgesia in the surgical field sufficient to produce this effect with great safety.

Chapter 4 of this volume deals with acupuncture-anesthesia and demonstrates that its application must be based upon a sound general knowledge of, and accomplished skill in, acupuncture. The study of surgery would be unthinkable and the results disastrous without a solid foundation in anatomy, physiology and other basic disciplines. Similarly precarious would be the attempt to go into acupuncture-anesthesia without a thorough understanding and adequate skill in the entire field of acupuncture, qualifications which cannot be acquired in a quick "crash course." They demand extensive instruction, as the Chinese acupuncturists receive it, men or women, scientific physicians or "barefoot doctors."

For these reasons the authors of this book decided to base their work on selective translations from several modern books on acupuncture therapy, as it is currently used in the People's Republic of China.

EDUCATIONAL AND LEGAL DEVELOPMENTS

The imbalance between the general desire of the public for a broad access to acupuncture therapy and its scant availability on a professionally acceptable basis has stirred up considerable action in the United States, since our book was first published just three years ago. Professional organizations, societies, and institutes have sprung up in many places; books, journals, and other periodic publications have made their appearance, and the ranks of acupuncture practitioners have swelled in an unprecedented fashion. Little material change, however, can be discerned in the field of education and training in the ancient art. As heretofore, little more is available to the prospective student than the customary weekend courses, brief seminaries, workshops, and symposiums which are offered in ever increasing numbers; often they are expensive and on occasion border on the bizarre.* Needless to say, this kind of training addresses itself exclusively to participants with an adequate foundation in the health sciences. Facilities for systematic and formal instruction in acupuncture, however, have as yet not developed beyond a formative stage in this country.

On the other hand, the legal posture to this new medical phenomenon has demonstrably progressed. By now, practically all fifty states and the federal government, in one way or another, have taken legislative or administrative action, the latter originating mainly from the state licensing boards. At the original publication of our book, only California had dealt with the problem legislatively in Assembly Bill No. 1500 enacted in 1972, which at that time became a model for regulations providing for qualified participation of the nonlicensed acupuncturist. Similar rulings, however, did not follow everywhere. The remaining diversity—and it is considerable—in the legal measures of the various states was made the subject of a comprehensive review in *The Journal of Legal Medicine* in March 1974. But not more than a year later, so many new regulations were enacted or existing ones amended that a complete reexamination was published in the same journal in March 1975. Yet, even this review did not remain the last word for long.

In the multiformity of legal positions, one view is expressed in many of the rulings, although by no means in all: Acupuncture is practice of medicine, osteopathy, or dentistry, respectively, and as a consequence may be performed only under appropriate license. In general

* For example, Outward Bound Wilderness Seminar Series, Stamford, Connecticut, 1975.

this authorization does not extend to licencees of other therapeutical disciplines, and some states, for example, New York, Pennsylvania, Mississippi, and Oregon, have underscored this stand by trial and conviction of operators outside the medical profession proper who performed needling on patients. Also in New York, Maryland, Washington, D.C., and in other states, acupuncture clinics and offices were closed that were staffed or operated in violation of existing codes. Some were later reopened when the legal deficiencies were remedied. It would therefore follow that anyone who intends to enter the field would do well to familiarize himself first with the legal situation in his particular location. Such a precaution may be advisable even for the full-fledged licencee, because in some states performance of acupuncture is subject to additional rules, such as its restriction to research and in-hospital settings or to presentation of positive proof of prior special training in the art—not to mention record keeping for peer review, submission of research projects, and analogous formalities. Some codes prohibit acupuncture outright.

Initiated by Nevada's "Act Relating to Chinese Medicine," passed in 1973, a more concrete approach toward regulating acupuncture has been taken by an increasing number of state legislatures. In several newly enacted bills acupuncture is dealt with as a professional or learned occupation, either within the frame of Chinese medicine as a whole or as a separate entity. As such it is, with slight variations in the different states, regulated by rules that customarily govern professional fields: educational requirements, licensing procedures, professional ethics and conduct, disciplinary measures, and so on. At this writing such legislation is also in force in Hawaii, Florida, and California. The last state has thus developed its "interim" legislation of 1972 into the Moscone Bill, Senate Bill No. 86, which treats the entire project in a very comprehensive and equitable fashion that could again serve as a model.

All these bills and similar ones that may follow create a novel legal status: Acupuncture practice remains no longer the exclusive domain of the physician, osteopath, or dentist. A nonmedical acupuncturist licensed under, and performing within, the provisions of these laws is legally entitled to practice. In the majority of cases the rules provide for such acupuncture service on a referral basis and in this way are not unlikely to establish a position for the acupuncturist that will be similar to the various other professions ancillary to medicine. In time this will open up new careers, but that will require an educational process which starts at the beginning and offers the student all basic and clinical instruction necessary for a license in acupuncture. No such system, which belongs in schools of higher education, exists in this country at the present time.

Specific legislation, such as that described above, is reportedly pending in Maryland, Massachusetts, New Jersey, and South Carolina. In the interim, and in other states where no legislative steps seem to be contemplated, a rule should be kept in mind that classifies acupuncture as an "experimental procedure." This follows a "Notice" of the Federal Food and Drug Administration in the *Federal Register* (vol. 38, no. 46, 1973), which rules that equipment and drugs used in acupuncture be labeled "experimental." The ruling has been enforced in federal court on several occasions. It entails—and this is mandatory—that the user of such items in the treatment of patients secure their prior informed consent. In other words, the patient has to be given full understanding of the risk/benefit ratio of acupuncture as compared with other available treatments.

The newness of acupuncture in American health care together with its classification (by federal ruling) as experimental will also play a role in professional liability insurance practice. However, so far as can be determined at this time the insurance carriers have not taken a uniform stand on the coverage of acupuncture therapy in any of the healing disciplines, be it medicine, osteopathy, dentistry, and, especially, the newly emerging category of licensed acupuncturists. Yet, it can be safely stated that the chance of iatrogenic complications is actually rather remote, if and when acupuncture is administered by a well-trained practitioner. Generally, needle therapy will involve the patient in no more, and probably far less, risk than countless other therapeutic modalities. All this notwithstanding, a close check on the stipulations of their individual insurance policy is highly advisable for all who contemplate the practice of acupuncture therapy—more so now in the general turmoil that has developed in the coverage of malpractice.

As this new edition goes to press, the information available on the legal status with regard to the practice of acupuncture still presents a somewhat blurred image. Adding to the uncertainty is the fact that a number of state boards (medical, osteopathic, and particularly dental) have as yet not communicated a definitive position. Certain aspects of the whole complex may therefore remain temporarily undecided. All in all, a common denominator that has so far emerged in the regulation of acupuncture therapy on the state level is the requisite of a legal license to practice, either medicine, osteopathy, or dentistry in general, or—where specific laws already exist—acupuncture in particular. Additionally, the entire field is covered by federal statute whereby acupuncture is termed an "experimental procedure" necessitating informed consent from the prospective patient. Up-to-date information on any other regulations, extant or up-coming, will rest entirely with the vigilance of the individual practitioner.

THE ESSENTIALS OF ACUPUNCTURE

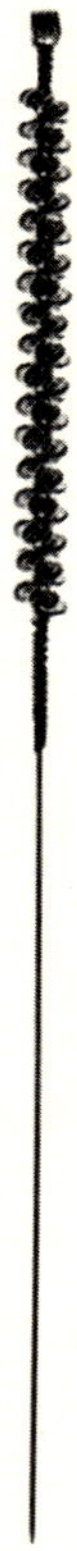

Fig. 1
Acupuncture needle

1 THE ESSENTIALS OF ACUPUNCTURE

The practice of acupuncture depends on acquaintance with the following features: acupuncture needles, techniques of acupuncture, moxibustion, electric acupuncture, and identification of acupuncture points. The practitioner must be familiar with the insertion of needles, the directions of needle insertion, responses to needle insertion, and methods of treatment.

ACUPUNCTURE NEEDLES

The two parts of a needle are its handle and its stem. The handle is made of either copper or aluminum while the stem is nowadays manufactured from stainless steel. The needles vary in length from 0.5 inches to 4.0 inches. The selection of the appropriate needle is dictated by the location of the acupuncture point. Needles 0.5 inches long are usually used for head and facial points, while needles 1.5 to 2.0 inches long are used for points located on the torso, arms, and legs. Needles 3.0 to 4.0 inches long are reserved for points situated in deep tissue or thick musculature, such as the glutei muscles.

Acupuncture needles also vary in diameter, from 26 gauge (0.45 mm) to 32 gauge (0.28 mm). Most frequently used are 30 gauge needles; for points around the eyes, 32 gauge; and for situations in which strong sensory stimulation is desired or for puncturing the skin to produce a drop of blood (blood-letting), 26 to 28 gauge.

TECHNIQUES OF ACUPUNCTURE

Insertion of needle. Preparation prior to acupuncture includes scrubbing the hands, prepping the site of insertion with alcohol, and examining the sterile needle for any defect. The two most popular techniques for inserting the needle are the following (see Fig. 2).

1. Using either the index finger or thumb of the left hand, digital pressure is applied to the site immediately adjacent to the acupuncture point. The handle of the needle is held between the thumb and index finger of the right hand while the third and fourth fingers support the stem. The needle is then directed towards the acupuncture point. By applying gentle pressure and continuously twirling the handle of the needle simultaneously, the needle is inserted through the skin at the acupuncture point to the depth desired.
2. An alternative technique, which is preferred for inserting needles of 3.0 inches or longer, is the following: holding the distal end of the needle between the thumb and index finger of the right hand, apply digital pressure to the site immediately adjacent to the acupuncture point with the left thumb or index finger, and then, with a jab, insert the needle through the skin at the acupuncture point. Next, after changing hands to support the stem of the needle with the left index finger and thumb, the needle is advanced to the proper depth by applying pressure and continuously twirling its handle with the index finger and thumb of the right hand.

Certain maneuvers may facilitate needle insertion when the following anatomical features are encountered. At locations where little musculature is present, one may pick up the skin and subcutaneous tissue with the fingers of the left hand for inserting the needle (Fig. 2). In addition, skin that hangs loosely or is wrinkled is stretched taut before inserting the needle into it.

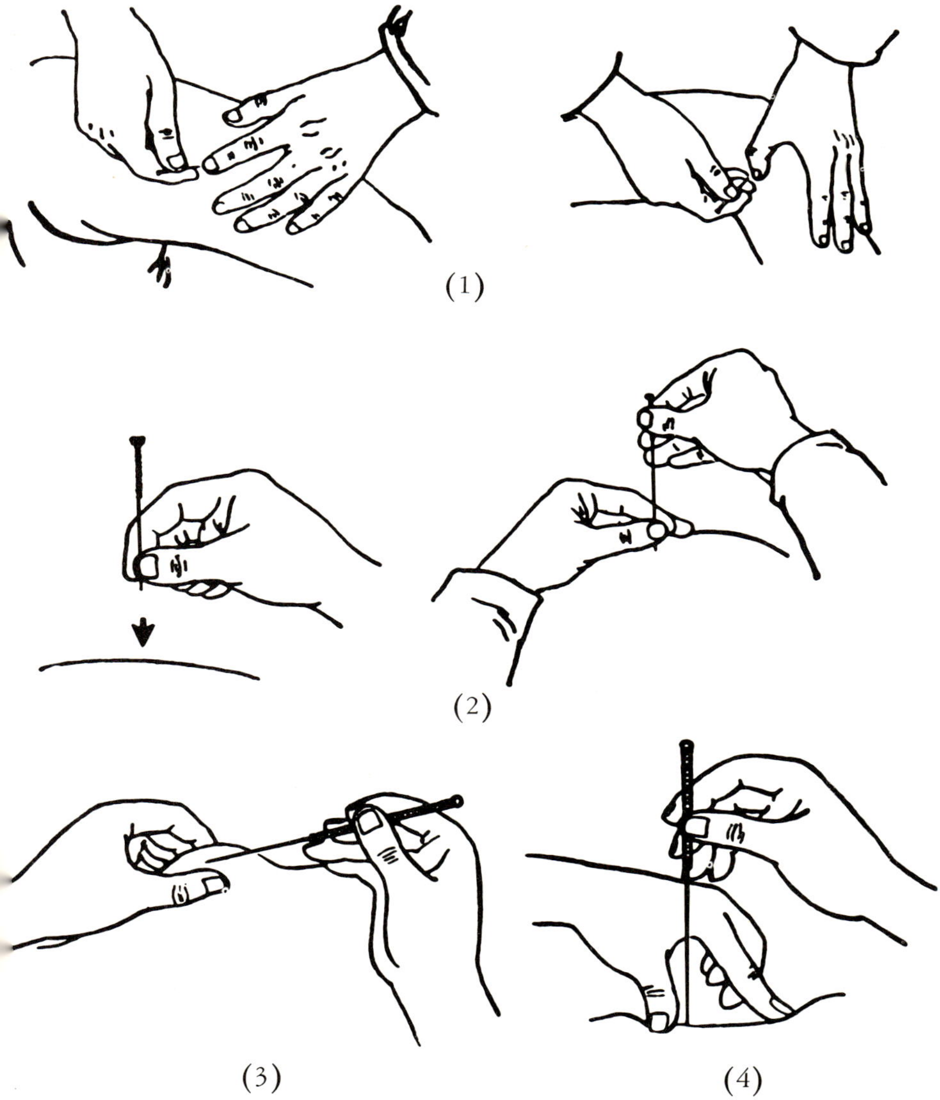

Fig. 2
Techniques of needle insertion

Directions of needle insertion (Fig. 3). Accurate insertion of the needle, with reference to direction, angle, and depth, must be achieved in order to produce safe and effective results. The directions and angles of insertion are as follows:

1. Perpendicular insertion. The needle and the skin at the acupuncture point should form an angle of approximately 90 degrees. This angle of insertion is generally used for deep insertion of the needle.
2. Diagonal insertion. The needle and the skin form an angle of between 30 and 60 degrees. This angle is also mostly used for deep insertion.
3. Horizontal insertion. The needle and the skin should form an angle of between 10 and 20 degrees. This is the usual angle of insertion at locations with minimal subcutaneous tissue or musculature.

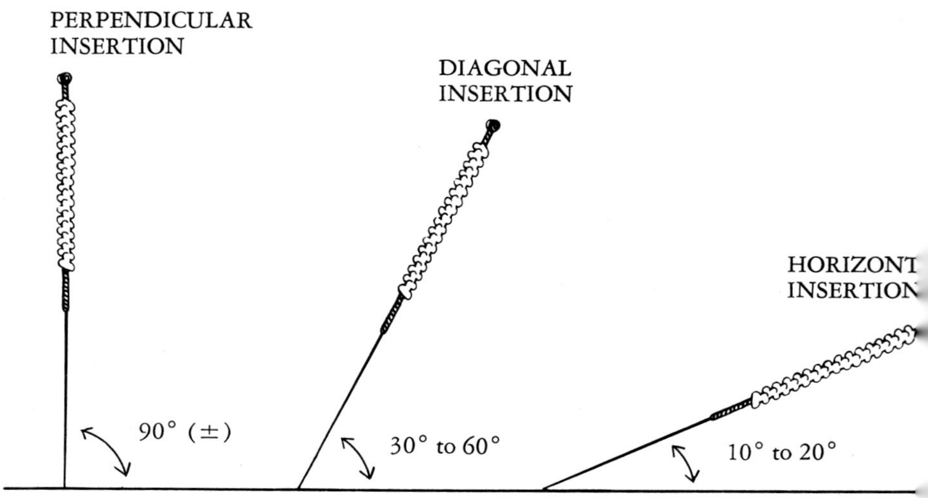

Fig. 3
Directions of needle insertion

The depth to which a needle is to be inserted is singular to each acupuncture point and is described in chapter 2. In general, a sensory response will be evoked from the patient when the needle reaches the appropriate depth.

Responses to successful needle insertions. Acupuncture, successfully executed, will elicit a variety of sensory responses from the patient. These range from a feeling of numbness at the acupuncture point to a sense of heaviness, dull ache, or tingling sensation which may be localized or radiating. These responses are known in Chinese as *Te-ch'i* 得氣 ("acquiring vital energy"). Puncturing of points on the head or face generally furnishes a sensation of heaviness or fullness; points located in deep musculature, numbness or a tingling sensation; while puncturing points at the fingertips usually produces a painful sensation.

Methods of treatment. The following methods are usually employed.

1. Short course therapy. Following correct positioning of the needle, as evidenced by appropriate sensory response from the patient, the needle is continuously twirled or agitated rapidly with an up-and-down motion for 10 to 20 seconds and then removed.
2. Intermittent therapy. The needle is twirled for several seconds intermittently with rest periods of a few minutes in between.
3. Continuous therapy. The needle is continuously twirled for several minutes or hours, or until symptomatic relief is obtained.

At the conclusion of treatment, the needle is removed by applying counterpressure on the skin adjacent to the needle with the left index finger as the needle is withdrawn while slowly twirling it with the right index finger and thumb.

Course of therapy. In general, acute conditions may be treated one to three times a day. Chronic diseases, however, are treated once every one to three days for a total of 10 to 20 treatments. This constitutes one course of therapy and it may be repeated after a rest period of one to two weeks.

MOXIBUSTION

Moxibustion—the application of heat to acupuncture points by burning *ai* or moxa, the dried leaves of *Artemesia vulgaris*—is used by itself or to complement acupuncture in the treatment of diseases. Heat can be applied directly by burning small cones of moxa at specific acupuncture points or indirectly by (1) heating an inserted needle with an ignited moxa cigarette (moxa rolled up in tissue paper like a cigarette), (2) holding the moxa cigarette approximately 0.5 inches above the acupuncture point when a needle is not used, or (3) heating a small pile of moxa on a slice of ginger placed over the acupuncture point. Treatment may be carried out for 10 to 20 minutes. Moxibustion is not recommended for facial points, superficial points that are in close vicinity to blood vessels, and points on the abdomen and back of pregnant women. It is, however, most effective in relieving arthralgias and abdominal pain.

ELECTRIC ACUPUNCTURE

A modality of recent origin, the utilization of an electric current for stimulation of an inserted needle is now widely and routinely employed in the practice of acupuncture. This innovation provides the following advantages:

1. It effectively replaces stimulation by manual twirling which can be quite fatiguing when treatment is prolonged.
2. The degree of stimulation can be accurately and evenly adjusted.
3. A stronger degree of stimulation can be achieved than by manual twirling.

Technique: Two acupuncture points must be used for each set of electrical leads, one for the positive and the other for the negative lead. These points should be located on the same side of the body, preferably in close proximity to each other. Connection of electrical leads to needles inserted at directly or diagonally opposite points of the body must be avoided in order to obviate the possibility of cardiac arrhythmias occurring from electrical stimulation. Following successful insertion of the needles, as evidenced by the proper sensory response, each needle is connected to one of the leads which in turn are attached to a direct current 9-volt battery power unit. The power unit is then turned on, the frequency of stimulation set, and the electric current slowly increased to a level comfortably tolerated by the patient. The frequency of stimulation is variable, ranging from as slow as 50 to 60 cycles per minute to as rapid as 100 to 200 cycles per second. The range most frequently employed is between 120 to 200 cycles per minute. As with manual twirling, a variety of responses such as paresthesia, numbness, a sense of fullness or heaviness, or a mild degree of muscle spasm will be elicited when the optimum amount of electric stimulation is administered. During the course of treatment, the patient's threshold of tolerance to the stimulation usually increases. Consequently, his sensory responses will be diminished. When this occurs, it will be necessary to increase the electric output to reestablish an effective degree of stimulation. Continuously increasing the electric current, however, may not be desirable and can be avoided by continually varying the output of the current, thereby preventing the patient from developing a tolerance to the stimulation. As a rule, acupuncture points on the face and below the elbow and the knee are more sensitive to electric stimulation than are points located elsewhere on the body.

Electric acupuncture is usually applied for approximately 10 minutes but this duration may be extended to four or five hours without producing any known ill-effects. Caution, however, must be exercised when using this form of treatment on patients with cardiac diseases.

POSSIBLE COMPLICATIONS OF ACUPUNCTURE

Complications from acupuncture, though infrequent, can nevertheless occur, especially when it is incorrectly practiced.

Formation of foreign-body granulomas may be provoked when

parts of the needle, fragile as it is, remain in the tissue after breakage. Such accidents may result from too forceful an insertion or withdrawal and from improper angulation or over-bending of the needle. As in the case of venipuncture or any other form of needle insertion, apprehensive patients receiving acupuncture may experience dizziness or even syncope.

Asepsis in technique, properly observed, should eliminate the possibilities of infection and hepatitis. An ill-advised or inadvertent insertion of the needle into the peritoneal cavity with subsequent injury to the organs therein may theoretically cause peritonitis and/or hemoperitoneum, even though this rarely occurs in practice. Ecchymoses at sites of acupuncture are not uncommon. They are more often seen with acupuncture-anesthesia when the needles are usually stimulated continuously for long periods. The ecchymoses essentially are of no clinical significance. However, serious bleeding may ensue from inadvertent needling of vital organs or major blood vessels. Similarly, pneumothorax and hemothorax are potential hazards associated with acupuncture in the region of the thorax. The insertion of needles into the central nervous system is also to be avoided when performing acupuncture at points along the vertebral column as transient paralysis may result from strong stimulation of the central nervous system.

IDENTIFICATION OF ACUPUNCTURE POINTS

Hundreds of acupuncture points have been documented in the Chinese literature of various periods. The majority of these points are located in linear arrangement along the major "meridians" of the body, of which twelve major pairs plus two at the midline of the body, front and back, have been established by tradition. Thus, except for the points situated along the midline meridians, each acupuncture point is paired, its companion point being located in a mirror-image position.

During the course of an ailment, localized pain may be elicited by applying digital pressure on certain points of the body. These tender spots, which are known as "pressure points," are also used as acupuncture points. Although the locations of these pressure points are not specific, they are usually found in the vicinity of the affected areas, as in the case of muscle spasms. However, they may also be located at a site distant to the afflicted organ, as exemplified by the acupuncture point for the treatment of appendicitis, Lan-wei-hsüeh, and the point for the relief of biliary colic, Tan-nang-hsüeh.

In the identification of a specific acupuncture point, reliance is placed on two systems.

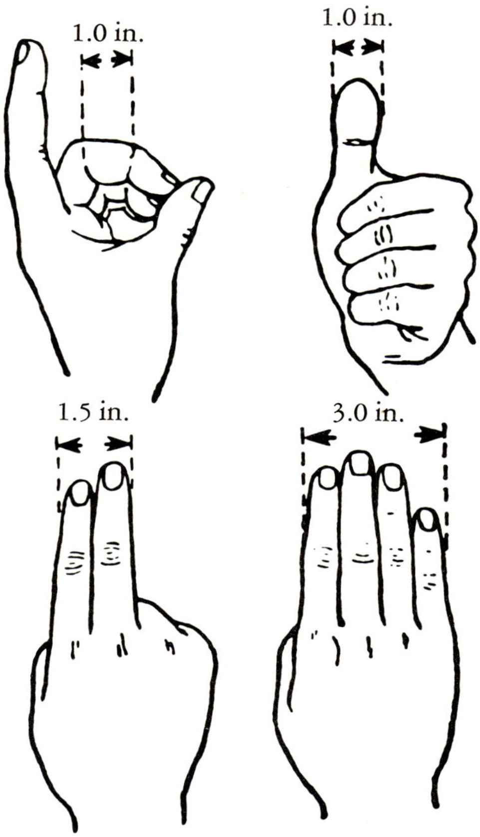

Fig. 4
Body-inch measurement

1. Body-inch method of measurement. One body-inch is equivalent to the distance between the joint creases of the interphalangeal joints of the patient's middle finger when it is flexed. It is also equivalent to the width of the patient's thumb. Furthermore, the total width of the patient's four fingers (excluding the thumb) measures up to 3.0 body-inches, while the combined width of the index and middle fingers is equivalent to 1.5 body-inches (Fig. 4). In this text, all inches mentioned in reference to the location of an acupuncture point are body-inches, which are specific for each patient.
2. Conventional anatomical landmarks such as easily identifiable bony structures, muscles, tendons, and external features.

MOST COMMONLY USED ACUPUNCTURE POINTS

2 MOST COMMONLY USED ACUPUNCTURE POINTS

The description of each acupuncture point covers its location in relation to conventional anatomical landmarks, indications for its use (diseases and symptoms amenable to treatment by stimulation of the acupuncture point in question), the recommended direction and depth of needle insertion, and a mention of moxa heating when its use will complement acupuncture. The last is not recommended when omitted in the text. When recommended, indirect heating is preferred.

The name of each acupuncture point is given in its transliterated version. In order to facilitate identification, an anatomical reference is ascribed to each point wherever possible, along with the organ specificity of the point. Each point is numbered within the section on points of that area of the body and the following abbreviations for the sections are used in cross-reference: HN for Head and Neck, UE for Upper Extremities, LE for Lower Extremities, CA for Chest and Abdomen, and B for Back. Thus, for example, HN–8 refers to Hsia-kuan, point 8 in the section on points of the head and neck.

POINTS OF THE HEAD AND NECK

1. Pê-hui, *vertex (Fig. 5)*

Location. At the vertex of the skull or at the point of intersection of a line joining the upper tips of the ears and a line drawn from the middle of the forehead directly towards the vertex.

Indications. Headaches, dizziness, syncope, hypertension, and rectal prolapse.
Technique. Horizontal insertion towards the front or the back of the skull to a depth of 0.5 to 1.0 inches.
Moxa heating. 5 to 20 minutes.

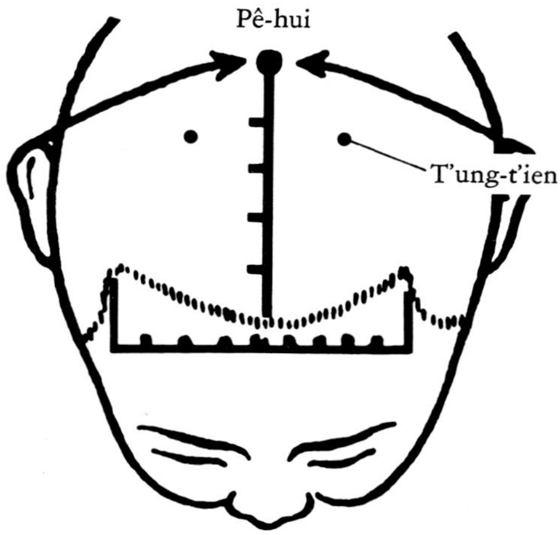

Fig. 5

2. T'ung-t'ien *(Fig. 5)*

Location. 1.5 inches lateral to a point 1.0 inches directly anterior to the point Pê-hui (HN–1).
Indications. Nasal infections (rhinitis, rhinorrhea), and headache.
Technique. Horizontal insertion anteriorly or posteriorly to a depth of 0.5 to 1.0 inches.
Moxa heating. 5 to 20 minutes.

3. T'ai-yang, *temporal (Fig. 6)*

Location. At the temple, at a point 1.0 inches directly posterior to the midpoint of a line joining the lateral canthus of the eye and the lateral margin of the eyebrow.

Indications. Temporal headaches, facial paralysis, tic douloureux, and eye diseases.
Technique. Perpendicular insertion 0.3 to 0.5 inches deep.

4. Yang-pê, *frontal (Fig. 7)*

Location. At a point one-third the distance of a line drawn directly upwards from the midpoint of the eyebrow to the hairline.
Indications. Facial paralysis, frontal headache, night blindness, and glaucoma.
Technique. Horizontal insertion laterally or medially 0.5 to 1.0 inches deep.

5. Shuai-ku, *supratemporal (Fig. 6)*

Location. 1.5 inches directly above the superior margin of the ear.
Indications. Temporal headache.
Technique. Horizontal insertion anteriorly to a depth of 0.5 to 1.0 inches.
Moxa heating. 3 to 5 minutes.

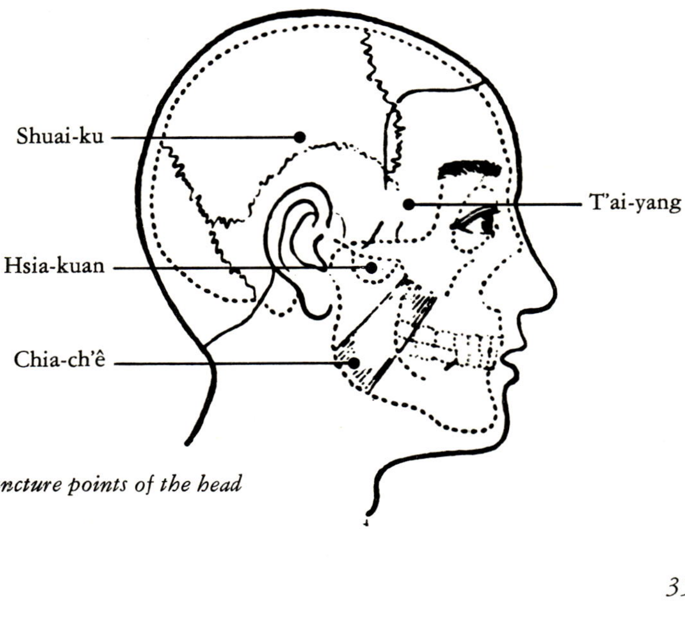

Fig. 6
Acupuncture points of the head

Fig. 7
Acupuncture points of the face

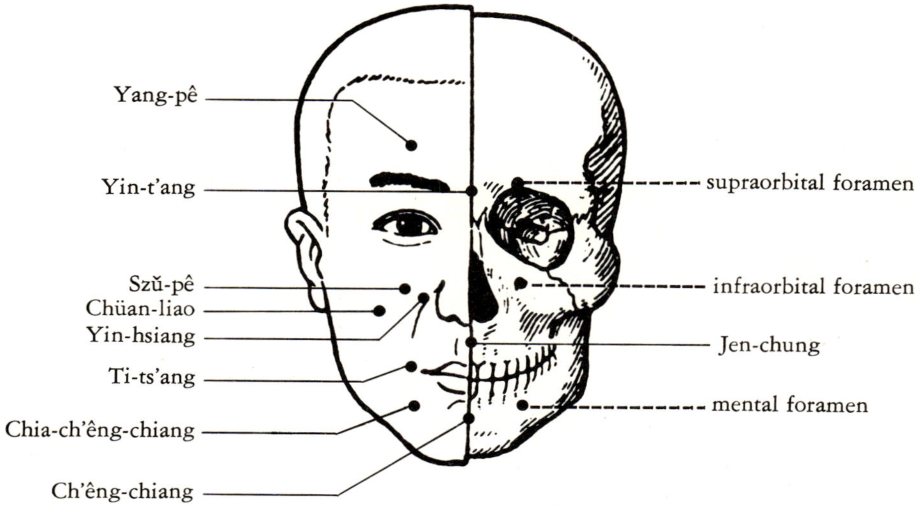

6. Yin-t'ang, *glabella (Fig. 7)*

Location. At the glabella, midway between the medial margins of the eyebrows.
Indications. Headache, dizziness, and nasal infections.
Technique. Horizontal insertion, caudad, 0.5 to 1.0 inches deep.

7. Szŭ-pê, *infraorbital foramen (Fig. 7)*

Location. At the infraorbital foramen or at a point one index finger's width directly inferior to the midpoint of the infraorbital margin.
Indications. Facial paralysis, tic douloureux, nasal infections, and eye diseases.
Technique. Perpendicular insertion 0.2 to 0.3 inches deep or horizontal insertion, caudad, 0.3 to 0.5 inches deep.

8. Hsia-kuan, *infratemporal fossa (Fig. 6)*

Location. In the infratemporal fossa, immediately anterior to the head of the mandible, or at a point one index finger's width anterior to the tragus of the ear. The head of the mandible can be easily palpated if the patient opens and closes the mouth.
Indications. Facial paralysis, tic douloureux, toothache, otitis media, and painful disorders of the mandibular joint.
Technique. Perpendicular insertion 0.3 to 1.5 inches deep, or diagonal insertion anteriorly or posteriorly to a depth of 0.5 to 0.8 inches, or horizontal insertion towards the corner of the mouth 1.5 inches deep.

9. Chia-ch'ê, *masseter (Fig. 6)*

Location. When the teeth are clenched, the point can be located in the body of the masseter muscle, one index finger's breadth anterior and superior to the angle of the mandible.
Indications. Toothache, facial paralysis, mumps, and spasm of the masseter muscle.
Technique. Perpendicular insertion 0.5 inches deep.
Moxa heating. 5 to 10 minutes.

10. Ching-ming, *medial canthus (Fig. 8)*

Location. With the eye closed, the point is 0.1 inches medial and slightly superior to the medial canthus of the eye.
Indications. Diseases of the eye.
Technique. Perpendicular insertion 0.2 to 0.6 inches deep. For treatment of myopia, the depth of insertion is 1.0 to 1.5 inches without any twirling of the needle.

11. Ch'êng-ch'i, *mid-infraorbital margin (Fig. 8)*

Location. Immediately superior to the midpoint of the infraorbital margin.

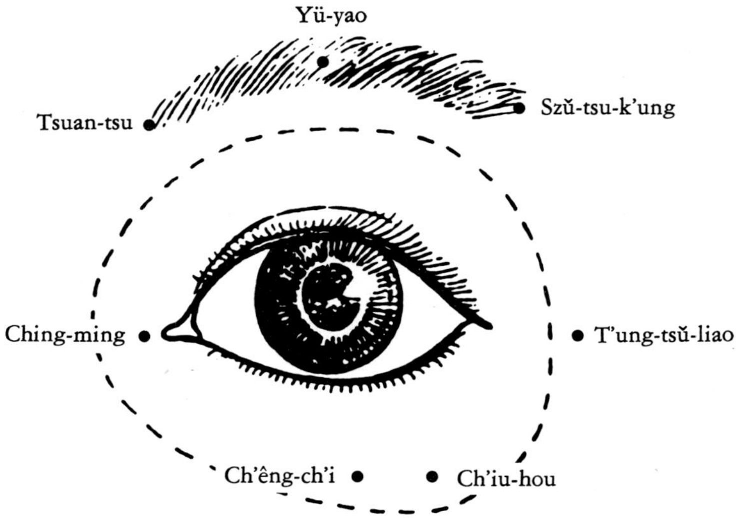

Fig. 8
Acupuncture points of the eye

Indications. Myopia and optic nerve disorders.
Technique. Perpendicular insertion 1.0 to 1.5 inches, with the patient looking upwards.

12. Ch'iu-hou *(Fig. 8)*

Location. Midpoint between the lateral border of the infraorbital margin and the point Chêng-ch'i (HN–11).
Indications. Optic nerve disorders, glaucoma, and myopia.
Technique. Perpendicular insertion 1.0 to 1.5 inches deep, with the patient looking upwards.

13. T'ung-tsŭ-liao, *lateral canthus (Fig. 8)*

Location. 0.5 inches directly lateral to the lateral canthus.
Indications. Diseases of the eye and headache.
Technique. Horizontal insertion posteriorly 0.5 to 1.0 inches deep.

14. Yü-yao, *mid-eyebrow (Fig. 8)*

Location. At the midpoint of the eyebrow.
Indications. Diseases of the eye.
Technique. Horizontal insertion laterally or medially 0.5 to 1.0 inches deep.

15. Tsuan-tsu, *superciliary arch (Fig. 8)*

Location. At the superciliary arch or medial margin of the eyebrow.
Indications. Diseases of the eye and headache.
Technique. Horizontal insertion, caudad, 0.3 to 0.5 inches deep, or perpendicular insertion 0.2 to 0.3 inches deep.

16. Szŭ-tsu-k'ung, *lateral eyebrow (Fig. 8)*

Location. At the lateral margin of the eyebrow.
Indications. Diseases of the eye and headache.
Technique. Horizontal insertion posteriorly or medially 0.3 to 0.5 inches deep.

17. Yin-hsiang, *nasolabial fold (Fig. 7)*

Location. At the superior aspect of the nasolabial fold.
Indications. Nasal congestion, rhinitis, and facial paralysis.
Technique. Horizontal insertion superiorly or caudad to a depth of 0.2 to 0.3 inches.

18. Jen-chung, *philtrum (Fig. 7)*

Location. At the philtrum and at a point one-third of the distance from the anterior nasal spine to the midpoint of the upper lip.

Indications. Syncope, epilepsy, shock, painful disorders and swelling of the face, and excessive salivation in children.
Technique. Horizontal insertion, superiorly, 0.3 to 0.5 inches deep.

19. Ti-ts'ang *(Fig. 7)*

Location. One index finger's breadth directly lateral to the corner of the mouth.
Indications. Facial paralysis, tic douloureux, and excessive salivation.
Technique. Horizontal insertion 0.3 to 0.7 inches deep, towards the angle of the mandible.
Moxa heating. 3 to 10 minutes.

20. Ch'êng-chiang, *symphysis menti (Fig. 7)*

Location. One index finger's width inferior to the mucocutaneous line of the lower lip at the symphysis menti, or below the midpoint of the lower lip.
Indications. Facial paralysis, toothache, and gingivitis.
Technique. Horizonal insertion, laterally, 1.0 to 1.5 inches deep.

21. Chia-ch'êng-chiang, *mental foramen (Fig. 7)*

Location. 1.0 inches lateral to the point Ch'eng-chiang (HN–20), at the mental foramen.
Indications. Facial paralysis and tic douloureux.
Technique. Perpendicular insertion 0.2 to 0.3 inches deep.

22. Êrh-mên, *superior tragus (Fig. 9)*

Location. Immediately anterior to the superior margin of the tragus of the ear.
Indications. Deafness, tinnitus, and otitis media.

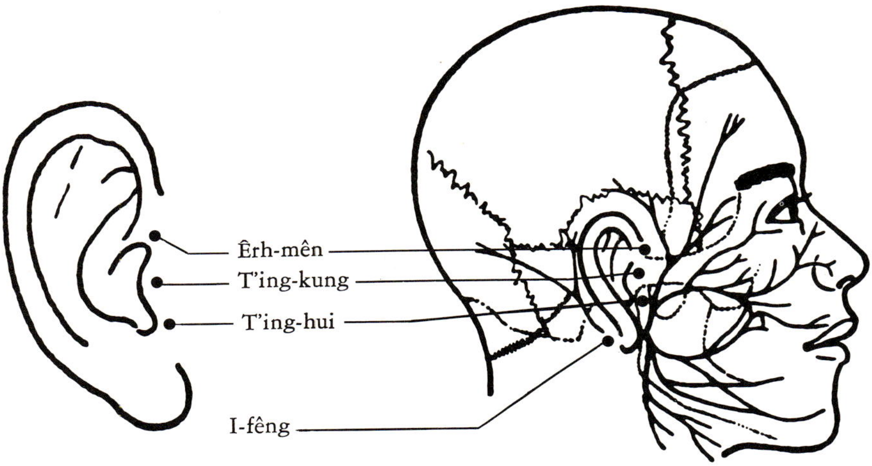

Fig. 9

Technique. With the patient's mouth open, perpendicular insertion 1.5 to 3.0 inches deep or diagonal insertion, caudad, to a depth of 2.0 to 3.0 inches.
Moxa heating. 3 to 5 minutes.

23. T'ing-kung, *mid-tragus (Fig. 9)*

Location. Immediately anterior to the middle portion of the tragus of the ear. Applying digital pressure on this point will occlude the external auditory meatus.
Indications. Deafness, tinnitus and otitis media.
Technique. With the patient's mouth open, perpendicular insertion to a depth of 0.3 to 1.5 inches.
Moxa heating. 3 to 5 minutes.

24. T'ing-hui, *inferior tragus (Fig. 9)*

Location. Immediately anterior to the inferior margin of the tragus of the ear.
Indications. Deafness, tinnitus, and otitis media.
Technique. With the patient's mouth open, perpendicular insertion, slightly posteriorly, to a depth of 1.0 to 2.0 inches.
Moxa heating. 3 to 5 minutes.

25. Fêng-ch'ih *(Fig. 10)*

Location. Midpoint of a line joining the tip of the mastoid process to the posterior midline, in the groove between the trapezius and sternocleidomastoideus.
Indications. Influenza, dizziness, headache, neck pain, hypertension, and tinnitus.
Technique. Diagonal insertion, medially and slightly caudad, 0.5 to 0.8 inches deep.
Moxa heating. 3 to 5 minutes.

26. Ya-mên, *C1–C2 (Fig. 10)*

Location. At the posterior midline, 0.5 inches above the hairline (between the first and second cervical vertebrae).
Indications. Mutism, deafness, occipital headache, torticollis, and mental disorders.
Technique. With the patient's head slightly flexed, perpendicular insertion, without any twirling motion, to a depth of approximately 1.0 inches. Successful penetration will elicit a localized sensation of pressure or fullness. However, should the patient experience paresthesia of all extremities, the needle should be immediately withdrawn.

27. T'ien-chu, *paravertebral C1–C2 (Fig. 10)*

Location. 1.5 inches lateral to the point for Ya-mên (HN–26) or

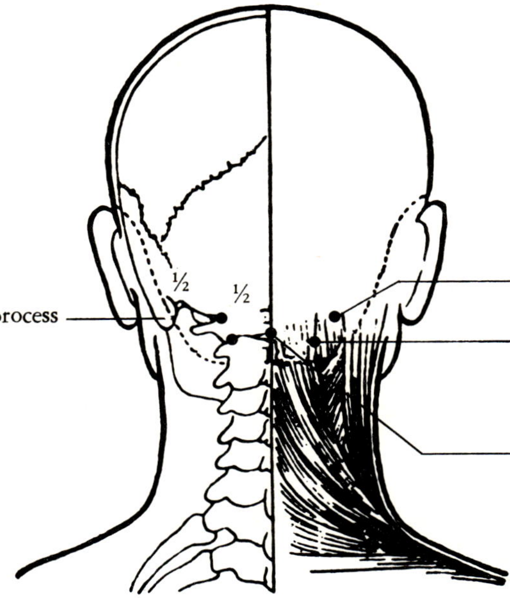

Fig. 10

at the lateral border of the insertion of the trapezius.
Indications. Occipital headache and torticollis.
Technique. Perpendicular insertion approximately 0.5 inches deep.
Moxa heating. 5 minutes.

28. I-fêng, *post-auricular (Fig. 9)*

Location. In the groove between the ear lobe and the mastoid process.
Indications. Deafness, tinnitus, otitis media, facial paralysis, and mumps.
Technique. Perpendicular insertion, slightly caudad, 0.5 to 1.0 inches deep.

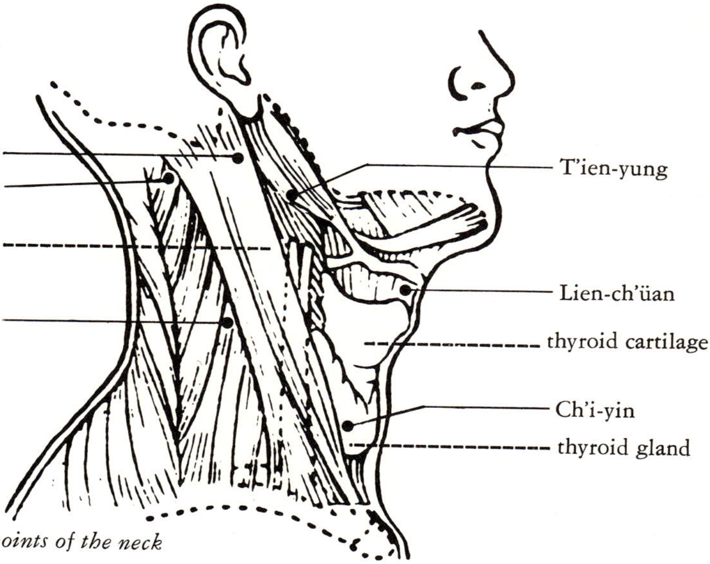

Fig. 11
Acupuncture points of the neck

29. I-ming, *mastoid process (Fig. 11)*

Location. Immediately below the tip of the mastoid process.
Indications. Tinnitus, myopia, optic nerve atrophy, cataracts, insomnia, mumps, and neurasthenia.
Technique. Perpendicular insertion 0.5 to 1.0 inches deep.

30. T'ien-yung, *mandibular angle (Fig. 11)*

Location. Immediately posterior and inferior to the angle of the mandible and anterior to the sternocleidomastoideus.
Indications. Tonsillitis, swelling and painful disorders of the neck.
Technique. Perpendicular insertion to a depth of 0.5 to 1.0 inches.
Moxa heating. 3 to 5 minutes.

31. T'ien-yu, *post-mastoid process (Fig. 11)*

Location. Immediately posterior and inferior to the mastoid process at the hairline or at the posterior margin of the insertion of the sternocleidomastoideus.

Indications. Tinnitus, deafness, torticollis, and pharyngitis.
Technique. Perpendicular insertion approximately 0.5 inches deep.
Moxa heating. 3 to 5 minutes.

32. Fuh-t'u, *mid-sternocleidomastoideus (Fig. 11)*

Location. 3.0 inches directly lateral to the laryngeal prominence of the thyroid cartilage at the posterolateral margin of the sternocleidomastoideus.
Indications. Hoarseness and dysphagia.
Technique. Perpendicular insertion to a depth of 0.3 to 0.5 inches.
Moxa heating. 5 to 10 minutes.

33. Lien-ch'üan, *supra laryngeal prominence (Fig. 11)*

Location. At the midline, immediately superior to the laryngeal prominence and inferior to the hyoid bone.
Indications. Numbness of the tongue, mutism, and dysarthria.
Technique. Perpendicular insertion approximately 0.5 inches deep.
Moxa heating. 3 to 5 minutes.

34. Ch'i-yin, *thyroid (Fig. 11)*

Location. In either lobe of the thyroid gland at the level of the cricoid cartilage.
Indications. Goiter.
Technique. Perpendicular insertion 0.5 to 1.5 inches deep towards the center of the lobe, but not beyond it.

35. Chüan-liao, *zygomatic bone (Fig. 7)*

Location. Directly below the lateral canthus and at the inferior border of the zygomatic bone.
Indications. Facial nerve paralysis and toothache.
Technique. Perpendicular insertion 0.2 to 0.3 inches deep.

SUMMARY OF ACUPUNCTURE POINTS OF THE HEAD AND NECK

LOCATION		NAME	COMMON INDICATIONS		SPECIFIC INDICATIONS
Head	Vertex	Pê-hui T'ung-t'ien	Diseases of head	Vertical headache	Pê-hui: Rectal prolapse, diseases of the brain T'ung-t'ien: Diseases of the nose
	Temporal	Shuai-ku T'ai-yang		Temporal headache	T'ai-yang: Eye disease, facial paralysis, tic douloureux
	Frontal	Yang-pê Yin-t'ang		Frontal headache	Yang-pê: Eye diseases, facial paralysis Yin-t'ang: Diseases of the brain and nose
Malar		Szŭ-pê Chia-ch'ê Hsia-kuan Chüan-liao		Diseases of the trigeminal nerve and facial nerve	Szŭ-pê: Diseases of the eye and nose Chia-ch'ê: Mumps, toothache Hsia-kuan: Diseases of ear, toothache Chüan-liao: Facial nerve paralysis, toothache
Eye		Ching-ming Ch'êng-ch'i Ch'iu-hou T'ung-tsŭ-liao Tsuan-tsu Yü-yao Szŭ-tsu-k'ung		Eye diseases	T'ung-tsŭ-liao and Szŭ-tsu-k'ung: Temporal headache Tsuan-tsu: Frontal headache

Nose		Yin-hsiang		Yin-hsiang: Diseases of the nose, facial paralysis
Ear		Êrh-mên T'ing-kung T'ing-hui I-fêng	Ear diseases	I-fêng: Facial paralysis, mumps
Mouth		Jen-chung Ti-ts'ang Ch'êng-chiang Chia-ch'êng-chiang	Diseases of mouth and teeth	Jen-chung: Syncope, salivation Ti-ts'ang: Salivation, tic douloureux Chia-ch'êng-chiang: Tic douloureux
Neck	Back	Ya-mên Fêng-ch'ih T'ien-chu	Diseases of back of neck	Fêng-ch'ih: Hypertension, tinnitus, dizziness, influenza Ya-mên: Mutism
	Side	I-ming T'ien-yung T'ien-yu	Diseases of side of neck	I-ming: Mumps, diseases of ear and eye, insomnia, neurasthenia T'ien-yung: Tonsillitis T'ien-yu: Diseases of ear and throat
	Front	Fuh-t'u Lien-ch'üan Ch'i-yin	Diseases of front of neck	Fuh-t'u: Dysphagia and hoarseness Lien-ch'üan: Mutism, numbness of the tongue Ch'i-yin: Goiter

POINTS OF THE UPPER EXTREMITY

1. Chü-ku, *claviculo-scapular spine angle (Fig. 12)*

Location. At the angle formed by the clavicle and the spine of the scapula.
Indications. Painful disorders of the shoulder.
Technique. Perpendicular insertion to a depth of 0.5 to 1.0 inches.
Moxa heating. 5 to 10 minutes.

2. Chien-yü, *pre-acromion (Figs. 13 and 14)*

Location. With the arm abducted to a horizontal position, the point is located in a small depression immediately anterior to the distal tip of the acromion.
Indications. Painful disorders of the shoulder and upper arm, and paralysis of the upper extremity.

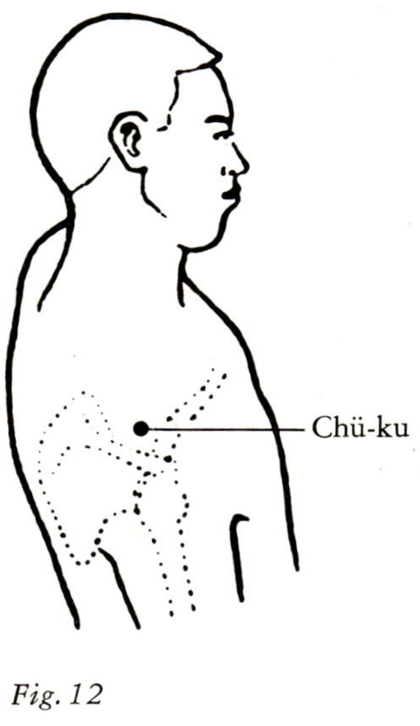

Fig. 12

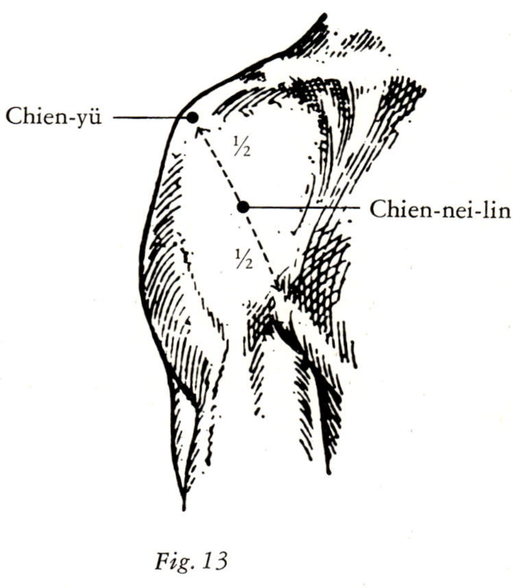

Fig. 13

Technique. After identification of the point and with the arm in a dependent position, perpendicular insertion, in a direction approximately parallel to the clavicle to a depth of 0.5 to 1.0 inches.
Moxa heating. 5 to 15 minutes.

3. Chien-nei-lin, *supra anterior axillary fold (Fig. 13)*

Location. Midpoint of a line between the point Chien-yü (UE–2) and the anterior axillary fold.
Indications. Painful disorders of the shoulder and upper arm, and paralysis of the upper extremity.
Technique. Perpendicular insertion 1.0 to 1.5 inches deep.
Moxa heating. 5 to 20 minutes.

4. Chien-liao, *post-acromion (Fig. 14)*

Location. In the depression immediately posterior to the distal tip of the acromion (easier to identify when the arm is abducted to a horizontal position).
Indications. Painful disorders of the shoulder and upper arm, and paralysis of the upper extremity.
Technique. Perpendicular insertion towards the axilla to a depth of approximately 1.5 to 2.0 inches.
Moxa heating. 5 to 20 minutes.

5. Nao-yü, *infra scapular spine (Fig. 14)*

Location. In the fossa immediately below the spine of the scapula and directly above the posterior axillary fold.
Indications. Painful disorders of the shoulder and upper arm, and paralysis of the upper extremity.
Technique. Perpendicular insertion to a depth of 1.0 to 1.5 inches.
Moxa heating. 5 to 20 minutes.

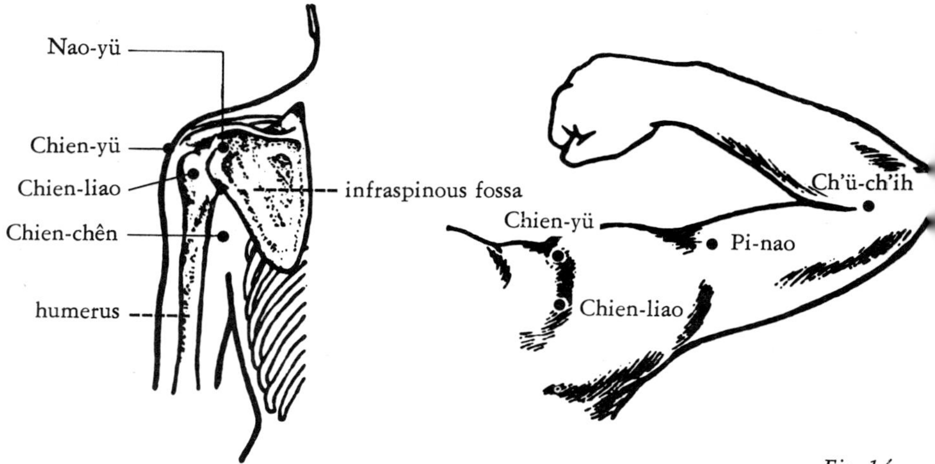

Fig. 14
Acupuncture points of the shoulder and upper arm

6. Chien-chên, *supra posterior axillary fold (Fig. 14)*

Location. 1.0 inches directly above the posterior axillary fold.
Indications. Painful disorders of the shoulder and upper arm, and paralysis of the upper extremity.
Technique. Perpendicular insertion to a depth of 1.0 to 1.5 inches.
Moxa heating. 5 to 20 minutes.

7. Ch'ü-ch'ih, *lateral antecubital fold (Fig. 14)*

Location. With the forearm flexed and abducted to a horizontal position, the point is located midway between the lateral epicondyle of the humerus and the lateral tip of the antecubital fold.
Indications. Painful disorders of the elbow and upper arm, paralysis of the upper extremity, fever, hypertension, neurodermatitis, pruritus, and other dermatological conditions.
Technique. Perpendicular insertion 0.5 to 1.5 inches deep.
Moxa heating. 5 to 20 minutes.

8. Pi-nao, *mid-humerus (Fig. 14)*

Location. With the forearm flexed and abducted to a horizontal position, the point is located immediately distal to the deltoid muscle, on a line joining the points Chien-yü (UE–2) and Ch'ü-ch'ih (UE–7).
Indications. Painful disorders of the shoulder and upper arm, and paralysis of the upper extremity.
Technique. Perpendicular insertion to a depth of 0.3 to 0.5 inches.
Moxa heating. 5 to 20 minutes.

9. Chi-ch'üan, *axilla (Fig. 15)*

Location. At the center of the axilla.
Indications. Painful disorders of the shoulder and upper arm, and paralysis of the upper extremity.
Technique. Perpendicular insertion to a depth of 0.5 to 1.0 inches.
Moxa heating. 5 to 10 minutes.

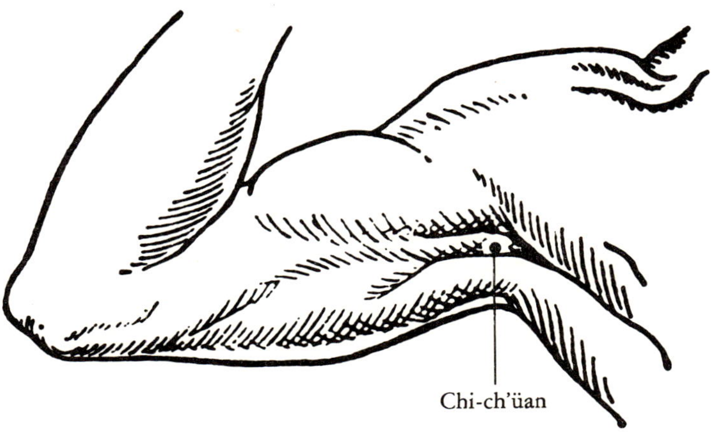

Fig. 15

10. Chou-liao, *distal humerus (Fig. 16)*

Location. With the forearm flexed and abducted to a horizontal position, the point is located 1.0 inches proximal to Ch'ü-ch'ih (UE–7) on a line drawn from Ch'ü-ch'ih to Chien-yü (UE–2).
Indications. Painful disorders of the elbow.
Technique. Perpendicular insertion along the ventral border of the humerus for a distance of 1.0 to 1.5 inches.
Moxa heating. 5 to 10 minutes.

11. Yang-ch'i, *anatomical snuffbox (Fig. 16)*

Location. With the thumb hyperextended, the point is located in the center of the depression bordered by the tendons of the extensor pollicis longus and brevis, and immediately distal to the styloid process of the radius (anatomical snuffbox).
Indications. Painful disorders of the wrist.
Technique. Perpendicular insertion to a depth of 0.3 to 0.5 inches.
Moxa heating. 10 to 15 minutes.

Fig. 16

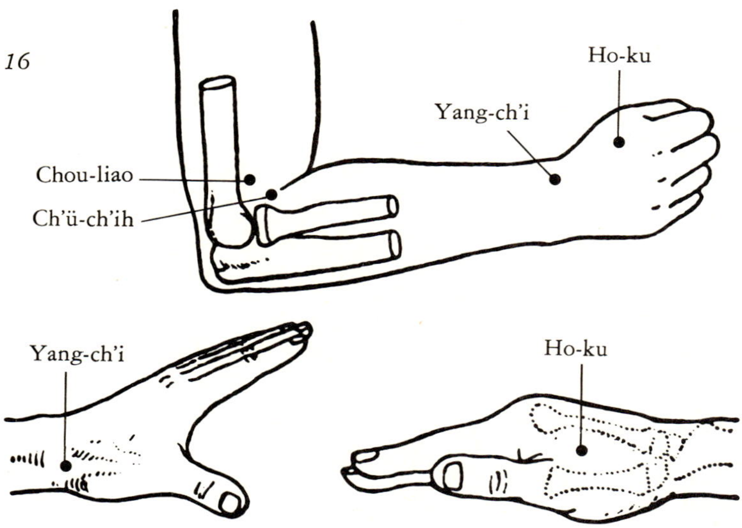

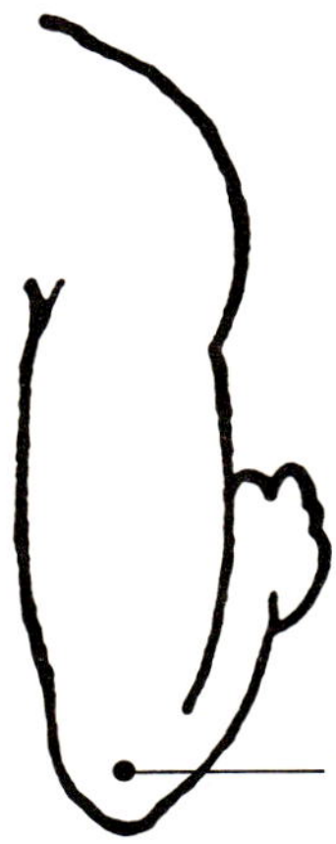

Fig. 17

12. Ho-ku, *first dorsal interosseous (Fig. 16)*

Do not use this point in pregnant women.
Location. At the midpoint of a line drawn from the web of the thumb to the confluence of the first and second metacarpals or at the proximal point of the crease formed by approximating the thumb and index finger. It can also be identified by pressing the entire distal phalanx of the thumb against the web of the patient's thumb and locating the point at the tip of the thumb.
Indications. Headache, toothache, pharyngitis, tonsillitis, rhinitis, sinusitis, tinnitus, deafness, eye ailments, induction of labor, menstrual cramps, goiter, painful disorders and paralysis of the upper extremity, neurodermatitis, arthralgia of the mandibular joint, and excessive perspiration.
Technique. With the hand resting on a table, perpendicular insertion to a depth of 0.5 to 1.0 inches.
Moxa heating. 5 to 15 minutes.

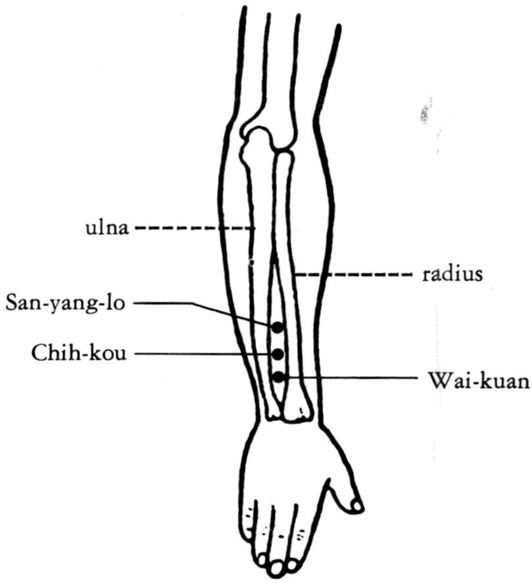

Fig. 18

13. T'ien-ching, *supra olecranon process (Fig. 17)*

Location. 1.0 inches directly proximal to the olecranon process.
Indications. Painful disorders of the elbow.
Technique. Perpendicular insertion 0.5 to 1.0 inches deep.
Moxa heating. 5 to 15 minutes.

14. Chih-kou, *dorsum of mid-forearm (Fig. 18)*

Location. On the dorsum of the forearm 3.0 inches proximal to the distal tips of the ulna and radius and between these bones.
Indications. Chest pain, shoulder and arm pain, and constipation.
Technique. Perpendicular insertion to depth of 1.0 to 1.5 inches.

15. Wai-kuan, *dorsum of distal forearm (Fig. 18)*

Location. On the dorsum of the forearm, 2.0 inches proximal to the distal tips of the ulna and radius and between these bones.
Indications. Paralysis of the upper extremity, chest pain, headaches, deafness, tinnitus, torticollis, and influenza.
Technique. Perpendicular insertion 0.8 to 1.5 inches deep.
Moxa heating. 5 to 15 minutes.

16. Yang-ch'ih, *dorsum, inter third and fourth metacarpals (Fig. 19)*

Location. On the dorsum of the wrist, in line with the confluence of the third and fourth metacarpals.
Indications. Painful disorders of the wrist.
Technique. Perpendicular insertion 0.2 to 0.3 inches deep.
Moxa heating. 5 to 10 minutes.

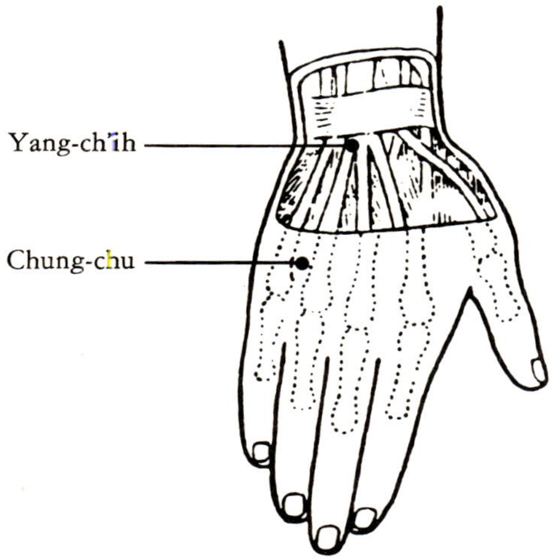

Fig. 19

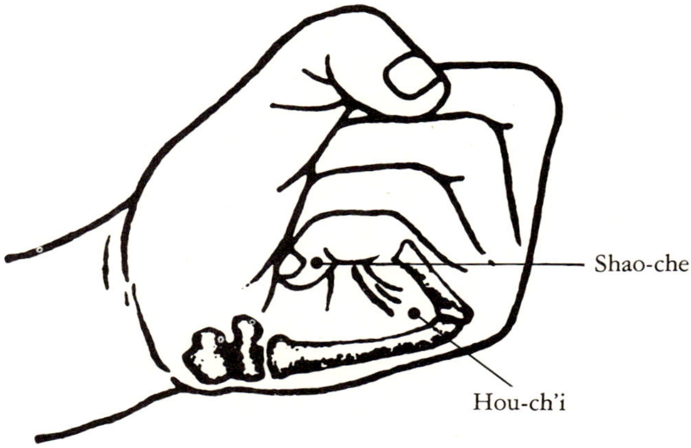

Fig. 20

17. Chung-chu, *inter fourth and fifth metacarpals (Fig. 19)*

Location. On the dorsum of the hand, between the fourth and fifth metacarpals and 0.5 inches proximal to the corresponding metacarpo-phalangeal joints.
Indications. Tinnitus, deafness, mutism, headaches, pharyngitis, and rigidity of the fingers.
Technique. Perpendicular insertion to a depth of 0.5 to 0.8 inches.
Moxa heating. 5 to 10 minutes.

18. Hou-ch'i, *distal fifth metacarpal (Fig. 20)*

Location. With the hand making a fist, the point is located at the medial tip of the major palmar crease, immediately ventral to the distal portion of the fifth metacarpal.
Indications. Occipital headaches, backaches, tinnitus, torticollis, and finger spasm and numbness.
Technique. Perpendicular insertion 0.5 to 1.0 inches deep.
Moxa heating. 5 to 15 minutes.

19. Shao-che, *fifth fingernail (Fig. 20)*

Location. At the intersection of the base and the ulnar margin of the fingernail of the fifth finger.
Indications. Insufficiency of lactation, mastitis, and headaches.
Technique. Diagonal insertion toward the interphalangeal joint to a depth of 0.1 inches.
Moxa heating. 5 to 15 minutes.

20. Ch'ih-che, *antecubital fossa (Fig. 21)*

Location. In the antecubital fossa immediately lateral to the tendon of the biceps. The point is best identified with the forearm in slight flexion.
Indications. Painful disorders of the elbow, cough, and pharyngitis.
Technique. Perpendicular insertion 0.5 to 1.0 inches deep.
Moxa heating. 5 to 10 minutes.

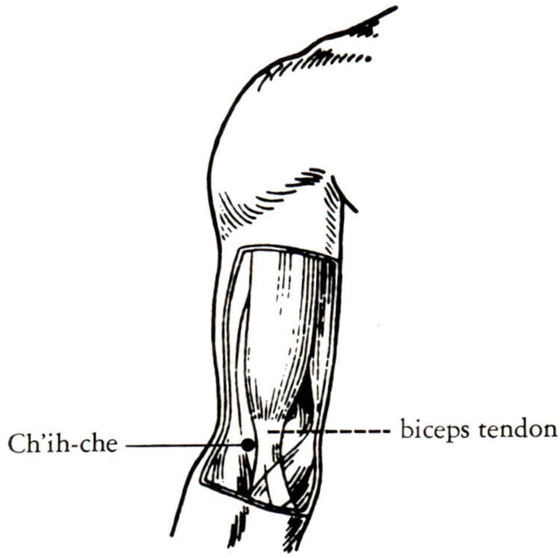

Fig. 21

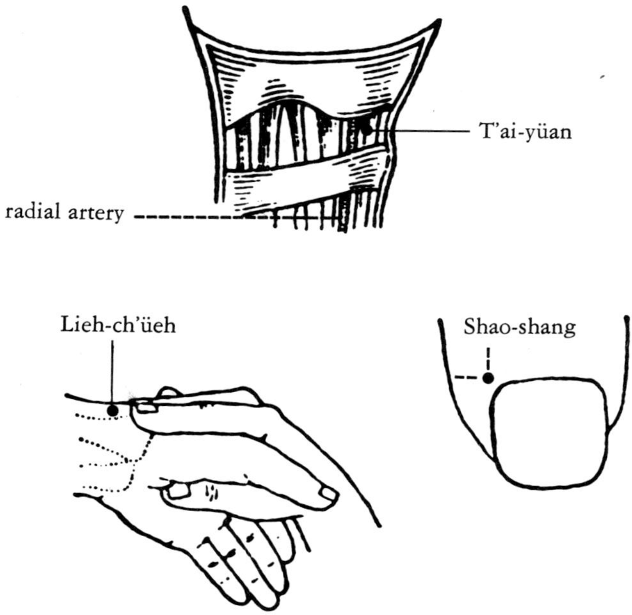

Fig. 22

21. Lieh-ch'üeh, *proximal to styloid process of radius (Fig. 22)*

Location. Immediately proximal to the styloid process of the radius or 2 fingers' width proximal to the anatomical snuffbox (see Yang-ch'i, UE–11) between the tendons of the abductor pollicis longus and the brachioradialis. It can also be located at the tip of the index finger of the opposite hand when the webs between the thumb and index finger of both hands are interlocked.

Indications. Painful disorders of the wrist, cough, and headache of the vertex of the head.

Technique. Diagonal insertion in the direction of the elbow, 0.5 to 1.0 inches deep.

22. T'ai-yüan, *lateral ventral wrist (Fig. 22)*

Location. Between the tendon of the abductor pollicis longus and the radial artery, at the level of the most distal crease on the ventral surface of the wrist.
Indications. Painful disorders of the wrist, cough, dypsnea, and pharyngitis.
Technique. Perpendicular insertion 0.2 to 0.3 inches deep.

23. Shao-shang, *thumbnail (Fig. 22)*

Location. At the intersection of the radial margin and the base of the thumbnail.
Indications. Cough, pharyngitis, tonsillitis, and syncope.
Technique. Diagonal insertion towards the base of the thumb 0.1 to 0.2 inches deep. This point is also for blood-letting in cases of syncope.
Moxa heating. 1 to 3 minutes.

24. Hsi-mên, *ventral forearm #1 (Fig. 23)*

Location. 5.0 inches proximal to the most distal crease of the wrist, on the ventral surface of the forearm and between the tendons of the flexor carpi radialis and palmaris longus.
Indications. Palpitations and angina pectoris.
Technique. Perpendicular insertion 0.5 to 1.5 inches deep.
Moxa heating. 5 to 15 minutes.

25. Chien-shih, *ventral forearm #2 (Fig. 23)*

Location. 3.0 inches proximal to the most distal crease of the wrist, on the ventral surface of the forearm and between the tendons of the flexor carpi radialis and palmaris longus.
Indications. Palpitations, angina pectoris, epilepsy, mental disorders, and malaria.

Technique. Perpendicular insertion to a depth of 0.5 to 1.5 inches.
Moxa heating. 5 to 15 minutes.

26. Nei-kuan, *ventral forearm #3 (Fig. 23)*

Location. 2.0 inches proximal to the most distal crease of the wrist on the ventral surface of the forearm and between the tendons of the flexor carpi radialis and palmaris longus.
Indications. Abdominal pain, epigastric pain, emesis, palpitations, angina pectoris, chest pain, numbness of the forearm and fingers, and malaria.
Technique. Perpendicular insertion 0.5 to 1.0 inches deep.
Moxa heating. 5 to 15 minutes.

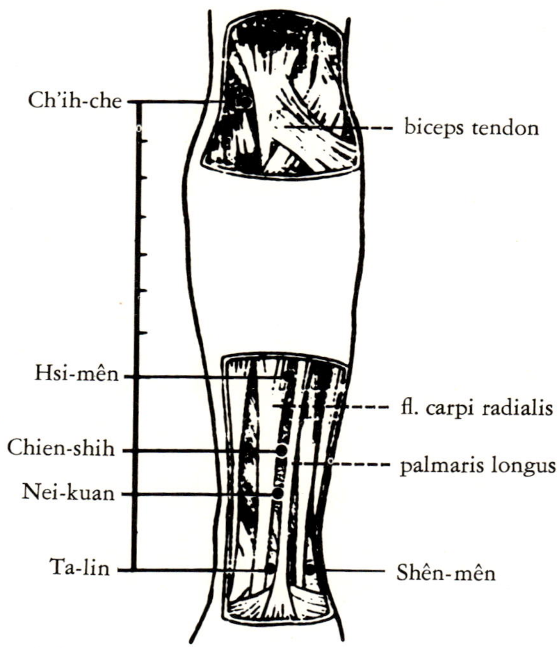

Fig. 23
Acupuncture points of the forearm, ventral surface

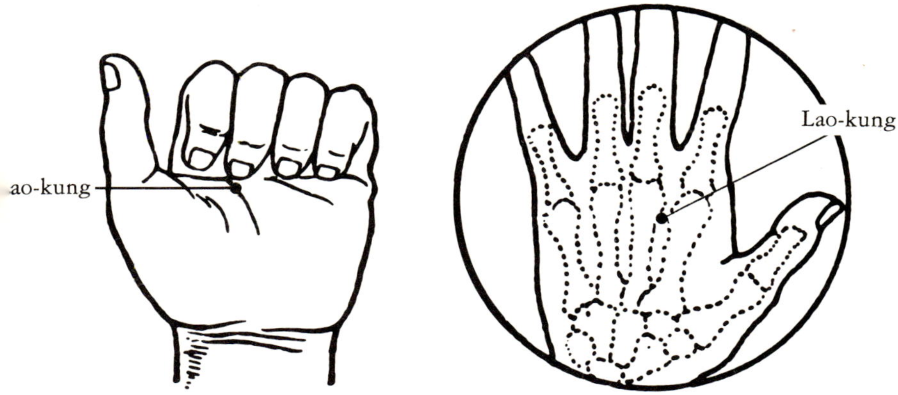

Fig. 24

27. Ta-lin, *midpoint of ventral wrist (Fig. 23)*

Location. Immediately proximal to the most distal crease on the ventral surface of the wrist and between the tendons of the flexor carpi radialis and palmaris longus.
Indications. Painful disorders of the wrist and palpitations.
Technique. Perpendicular insertion 0.3 to 0.5 inches deep.
Moxa heating. 5 to 15 minutes.

28. Lao-kung, *distal third metacarpal (Fig. 24)*
Location. On the palm, 1.0 inches from the third metacarpophalangeal joint, between the second and third metacarpals. It can also be located at the point where the tip of the completely flexed middle finger touches the most distal major palmar crease.
Indications. Dermatitis of the hand and stomatitis.
Technique. Perpendicular insertion 0.3 to 0.5 inches deep.
Moxa heating. 5 to 10 minutes.

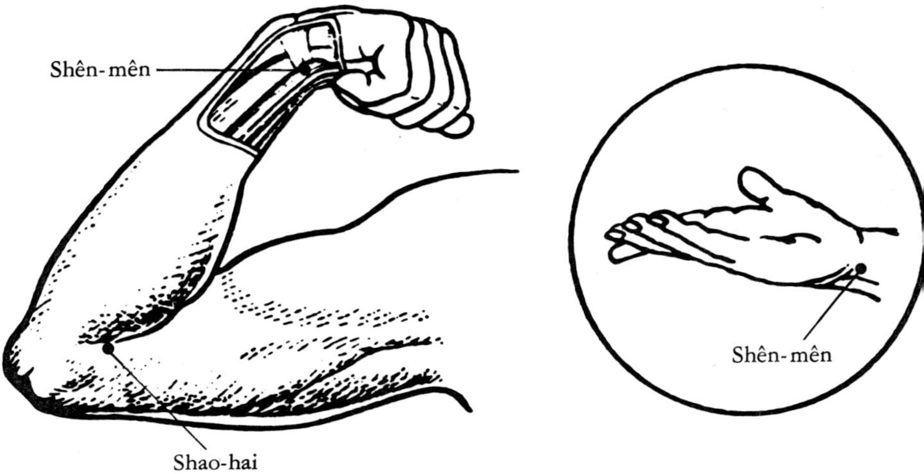

Fig. 25

29. Shao-hai, *medial antecubital fold (Fig. 25)*

Location. At the medial tip of the antecubital fold when the forearm is completely flexed.
Indications. Painful disorders of the elbow.
Technique. Perpendicular insertion 0.5 to 1.0 inches deep.
Moxa heating. 5 to 10 minutes.

30. Shên-mên, *medial aspect of ventral wrist (Fig. 25)*

Location. At the most distal crease on the ventral surface of the wrist, immediately proximal to the pisiform bone and medial to the tendon of the flexor carpi ulnaris.
Indications. Insomnia, palpitations, and neurasthenia.
Technique. Perpendicular insertion 0.3 to 0.5 inches deep.
Moxa heating. 5 to 15 minutes.

31. Pa-hsieh, *inter metacarpo-phalangeal joints (Fig. 26)*

Location. With the hand making a fist, the points are located 0.5 inches proximal to the webs of the fingers.

Indications. Painful disorders and numbness of the fingers and finger joints, headache, toothache, pharyngitis, and painful disorders of the neck.

Technique. With the hand loosely clenched, perpendicular insertion, parallel to the metacarpals, approximately 0.5 inches deep.

32. Shang-pa-hsieh, *inter distal metacarpals (Fig. 26a)*

Location. Between the distal portions of the metacarpals and immediately proximal to the metacarpo-phalangeal joints. The point between the first and second metacarpals corresponds to the point Ho-ku (UE–12) while the point between the fourth and fifth metacarpals is similar to the point Chung-chu (UE–17).

Indications. Painful disorders and numbness of the fingers and finger joints, headache, toothache, pharyngitis, and painful disorders of the neck.

Technique. Perpendicular insertion to a depth of 0.3 to 0.5 inches

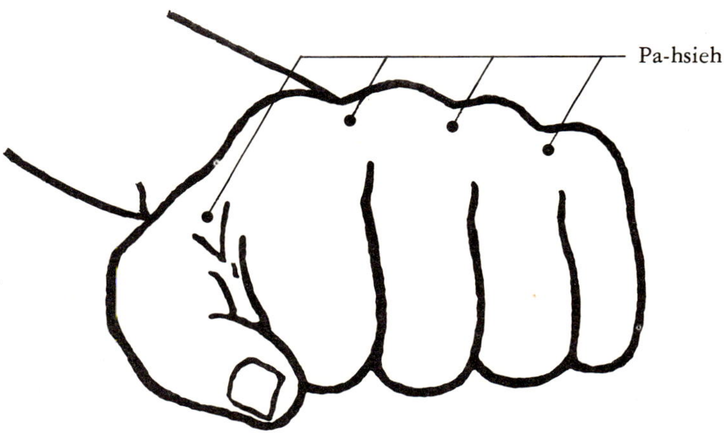

Fig. 26

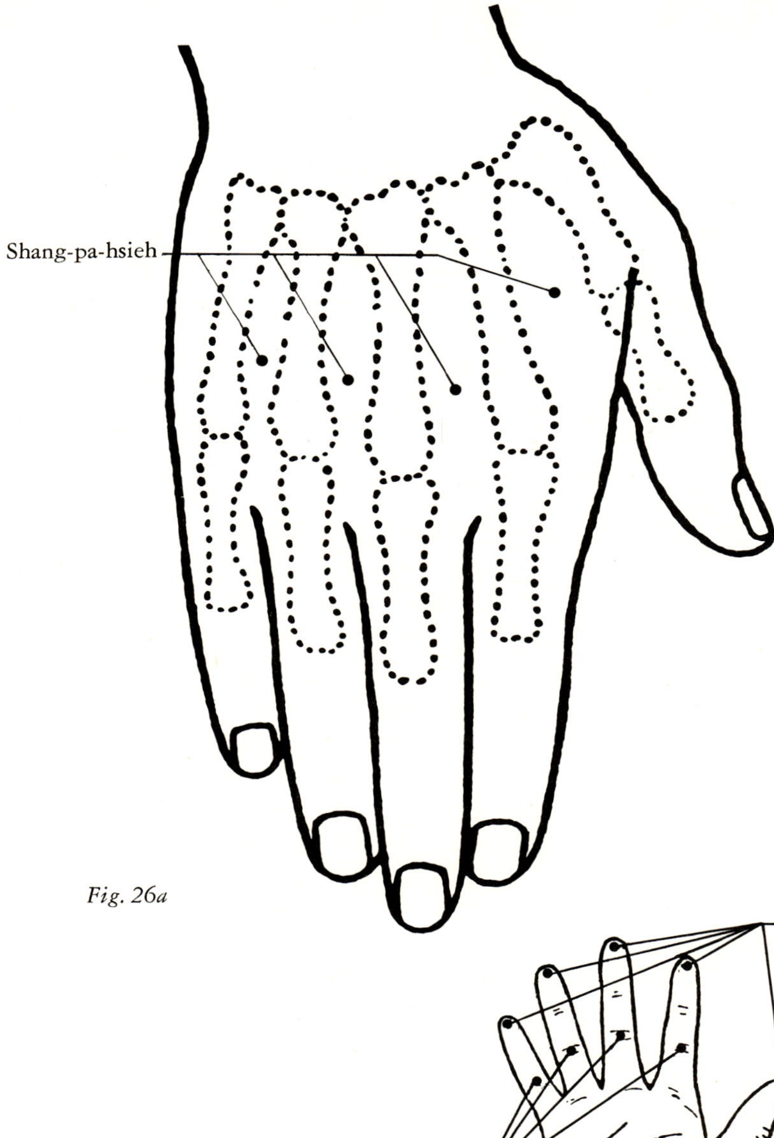

Fig. 26a

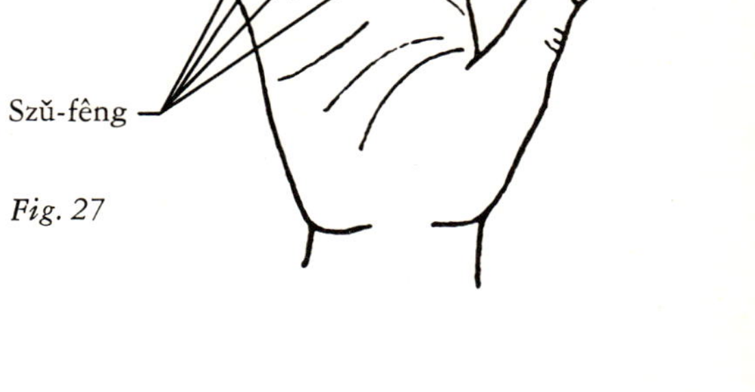

Fig. 27

33. Szŭ-fêng, *proximal interphalangeal joints (Fig. 27)*

Location. At the ventral surface of the second to the fifth proximal interphalangeal joints.
Indications. Pediatric digestive disorders and pertussis.
Technique. Perpendicular insertion 0.1 inches deep. This should produce the escape of a yellowish, transparent fluid.

34. Shih-hsüan, *fingertips (Fig. 27)*

Location. At the tip of each finger and 0.1 inches below the fingernail.
Indications. Syncope and shock.
Technique. Puncture each point till blood is produced (bloodletting).

35. San-yang-lo *(Fig. 18)*

Location. On the dorsum of the forearm, 4.0 inches proximal to the distal end of the ulna and radius and between these bones.
Indications. Deafness, laryngitis, and painful disorders of the arm.
Technique. Perpendicular insertion 0.5 to 1.0 inches deep.
Moxa heating. 5 to 20 minutes.

36. Kung-tsui *(Fig. 28)*

Location. 7.0 inches directly proximal to the point T'ai-yüan (UE-22).
Indications. Cough, asthma, tonsillitis, and pain and stiffness of the elbow joint.
Technique. Perpendicular insertion 0.5 to 1.0 inch deep.
Moxa heating. 3 to 10 minutes.

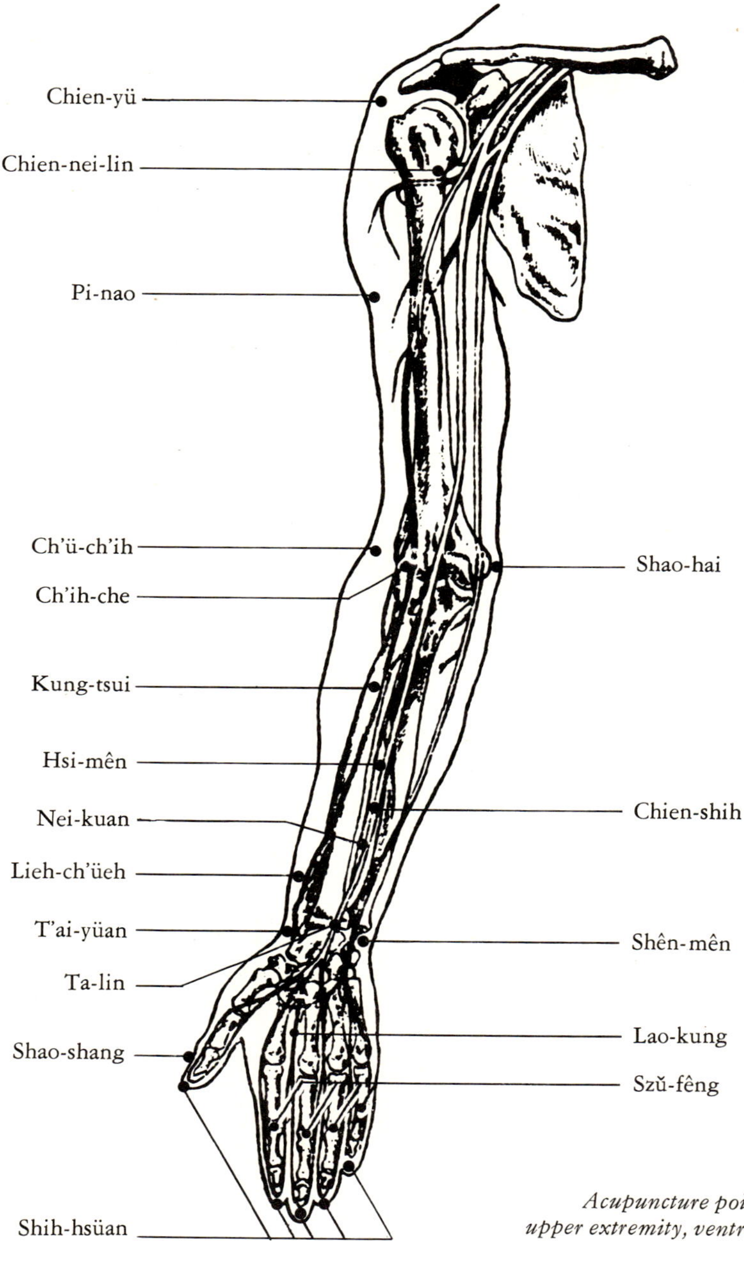

Fig. 28
Acupuncture points of the upper extremity, ventral surface

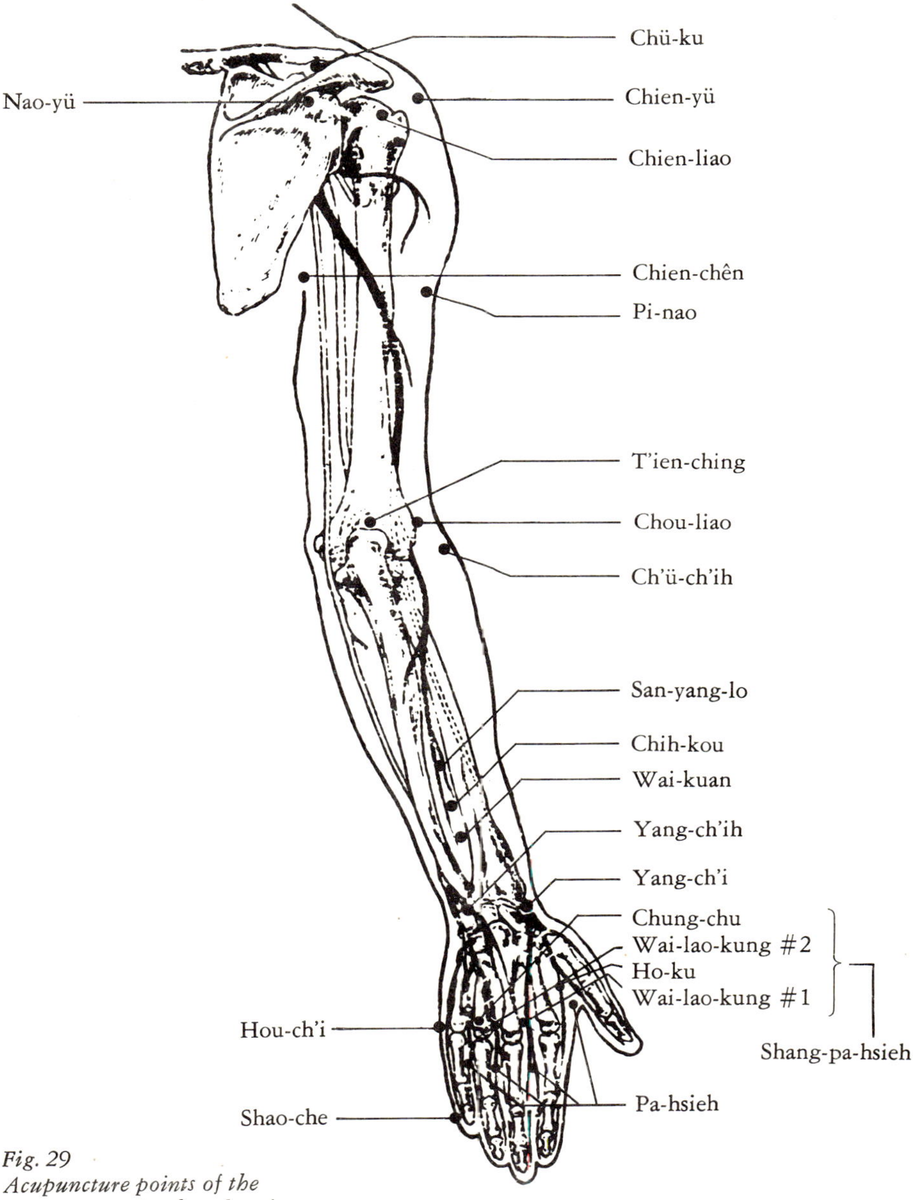

Fig. 29
Acupuncture points of the upper extremity, dorsal surface

Table 2

SUMMARY OF ACUPUNCTURE POINTS OF THE UPPER EXTREMITY

LOCATION	NAME	COMMON INDICATIONS		SPECIFIC INDICATIONS
Shoulder	Chü-ku Chien-yü Chien-nei-lin Chien-chên Nao-yü Chi-ch'üan Pi-nao		Painful disorders of the shoulder, paralysis of the upper extremity	
Arm and hand, dorsal surface	Chou-liao Ch'ü-ch'ih Yang-ch'i Ho-ku	Diseases of the head and throat	Diseases of the eye, ear, nose, and mouth	Chou-liao: Painful disorders of the elbow Ch'ü-ch'ih: Painful disorders of the elbow, hypertension, pruritus Yang-ch'i: Painful disorders of the wrist Ho-ku: Deafness, tinnitus, induction of labor, excessive perspiration, painful disorders of the mandibular joint
	T'ien-ching Chih-kou Wai-kuan Yang-ch'ih Chung-chu San-yang-lo		Diseases of the eye, malar, maxilla, mandible and chest	T'ien-ching: Painful disorders of the elbow Chih-kou: Constipation Wai-kuan: Torticollis, influenza Yang-ch'ih: Painful disorders of the wrist

	Hou-ch'i Shao-che			Hou-ch'i: Backache, finger spasm and numbness Shao-che: Diseases of the breast
Arm and hand, ventral surface	Ch'ih-che Lieh-ch'üeh T'ai-yüan Shao-shang	Diseases of the chest	Diseases of the throat and lung	Ch'ih-che: Painful disorders of the elbow Lieh-ch'üeh: Headache, painful disorders of the wrist T'ai-yüan: Painful disorders of the wrist Shao-shang: Syncope
	Hsi-mên Chien-shih Nei-kuan Ta-lin Lao-kung Kung-tsui		Diseases of the heart	Chien-shih: Epilepsy, malaria Nei-kuan: Painful disorders of the stomach and intestine, malaria Ta-lin: Painful disorders of the wrist Lao-kung: Stomatitis, dermatitis of the hand Kung-tsui: Cough, asthma, pain of elbow joint
	Shao-hai Shên-mên			Shao-hai: Painful disorders of the elbow Shên-mên: Insomnia
Hand, dorsum	Pa-hsieh Shang-pa-hsieh		Painful disorders and numbness of the fingers	
Hand, ventral surface	Szŭ-fêng Shih-hsüan			Szŭ-fêng: Pediatric digestive disorders, pertussis Shih-hsüan: Syncope

POINTS OF THE LOWER EXTREMITY

1. Huan-t'iao, *posterior hip (Fig. 30)*

Location. With the patient lying in a lateral position and with the knees partially flexed, the point is located at one-third the distance of a line drawn from the greater trochanter of the femur to the base of the coccyx.
Indications. Sciatica, paralysis of the lower extremity, and painful disorders of the hip.
Technique. Perpendicular insertion 2.0 to 3.0 inches deep.
Moxa heating. 10 to 30 minutes.

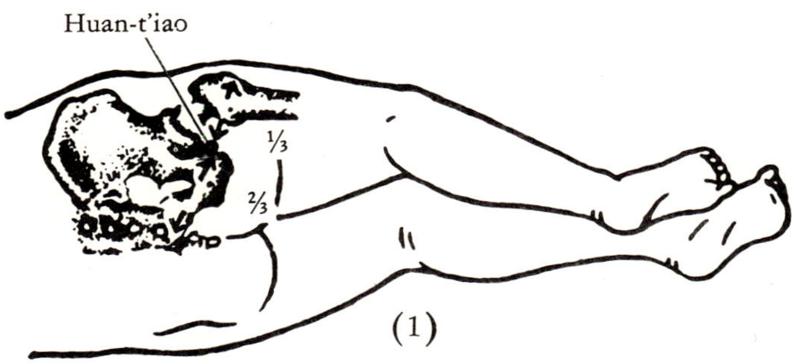

(1)

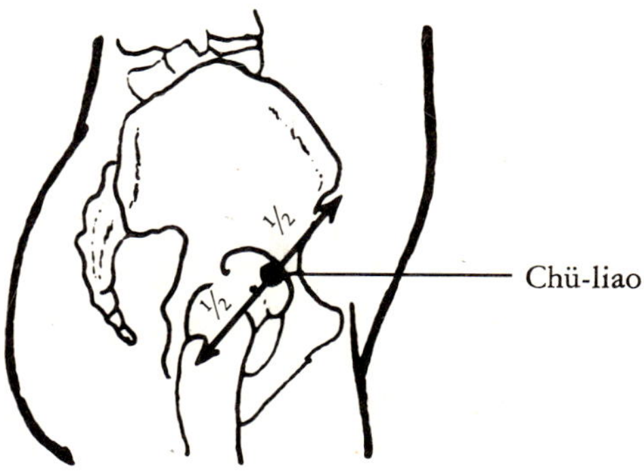

Fig. 30
Acupuncture points of the hip

(2)

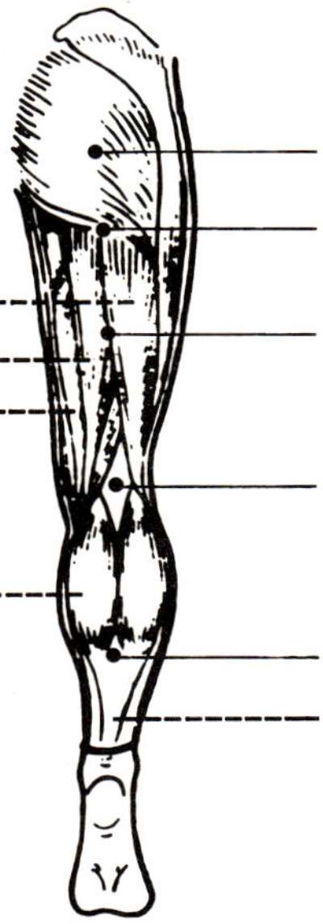

Fig. 31
Acupuncture points of the lower extremity, posterior surface

2. Chü-liao, *lateral hip (Fig. 30)*

Location. With the patient lying in a lateral position and with the knees partially flexed, it is at the midpoint of a line drawn from the anterior superior iliac spine to the greater trochanter of the femur.
Indications. Painful disorders of the hip and lower extremity.
Technique. Perpendicular insertion 2.0 to 3.0 inches deep.
Moxa heating. 5 to 20 minutes.

3. Ch'êng-fu, *gluteal fold (Fig. 31)*

Location. At the midline on the posterior surface of the thigh and at the level of the gluteal fold.
Indications. Sciatica, paralysis of the lower extremity, hemorrhoids, renal failure, and low back pain.
Technique. Perpendicular insertion 1.5 to 2.5 inches deep.
Moxa heating. 5 to 20 minutes.

4. Yin-lien, *base of femoral triangle (Fig. 32)*

Location. 1.0 inches distal to the inguinal ligament and immediately lateral to the femoral artery.
Indications. Low back pain, and paralysis and pain of the lower extremity.
Technique. Perpendicular insertion 1.0 to 1.5 inches deep.
Moxa heating. 5 to 10 minutes.

5. Fu-t'u, *anterior mid-thigh (Fig. 32)*

Location. On the anterior surface of the thigh, 6.0 inches directly proximal to the lateral edge of the base of the patella. The distance of the point from the base of the patella is equivalent to the length of the patient's hand.
Indications. Paralysis of the lower extremity and painful disorders of the knee.
Technique. Perpendicular insertion along the lateral edge of the femur to a depth of 2.0 to 3.0 inches.
Moxa heating. 5 to 20 minutes.

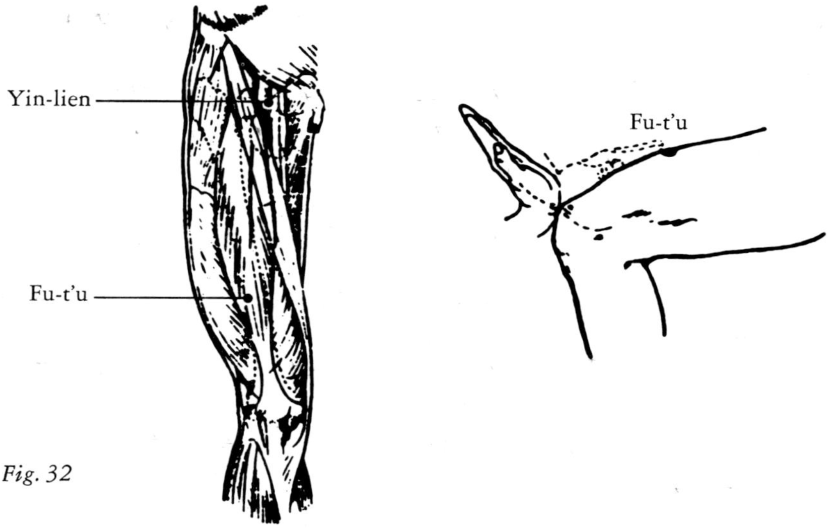

Fig. 32

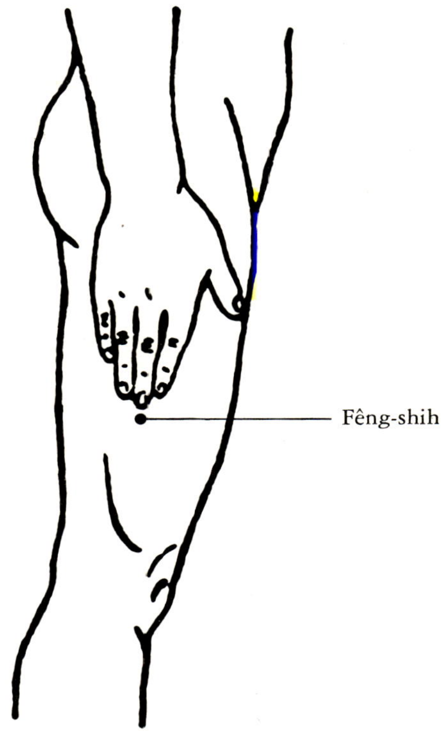

Fig. 33

6. Fêng-shih, *lateral mid-thigh (Fig. 33)*

Location. At the midline on the lateral aspect of the thigh, 7.0 inches directly proximal to a line at the level of the base of the patella. With the patient standing erect and his arm hanging at his side, the point can also be located immediately distal to the tip of the middle finger on the lateral surface of the thigh.
Indications. Paralysis and pain of the lower extremity, low back pain, and neurodermatitis of the lateral aspect of the thigh.
Technique. Perpendicular insertion 1.5 to 2.5 inches deep.
Moxa heating. 5 to 20 minutes.

7. Yin-mên, *posterior mid-thigh (Fig. 31)*

Location. At the midline on the posterior aspect of the thigh, 6.0 inches directly distal to the point Ch'êng-fu (LE–3) or to the gluteal fold.
Indications. Sciatica, lumbago, and paralysis of the lower extremity.
Technique. Perpendicular insertion 1.5 to 3.0 inches deep.
Moxa heating. 5 to 20 minutes.

8. Nei-wai-ch'i-yen, *para ligament patellae (Fig. 34)*

Location. In the joint space on each side of the ligament patellae.
Indications. Painful disorders of the knee.
Technique. Perpendicular insertion 1.5 to 2.0 inches deep.
Moxa heating. 5 to 15 minutes.

9. Liang-ch'iu, *supra lateral patella (Fig. 34)*

Location. 2.0 inches directly proximal to the lateral edge of the base of the patella.
Indications. Painful disorders of the knee, numbness of the lower extremity, and gastralgia.
Technique. Perpendicular insertion to a depth of 1.0 to 1.5 inches.
Moxa heating. 5 to 15 minutes.

10. Tsu-san-li, *pretibial #1 (Fig. 34)*

Location. 3.0 inches directly distal to the point where the lateral and apical (distal) margins of the patella meet. It can also be located at a point 1.0 inches distal and lateral to the tibial tubercle (tuberosity).
Indications. Abdominal pain, gastralgia, diarrhea, gastro-intestinal complaints, hypertension, malaise, fatigue, anemia, paralysis of the lower extremity, and painful disorders of the knee.
Technique. Perpendicular insertion 1.0 to 2.0 inches deep.
Moxa heating. 10 to 30 minutes.

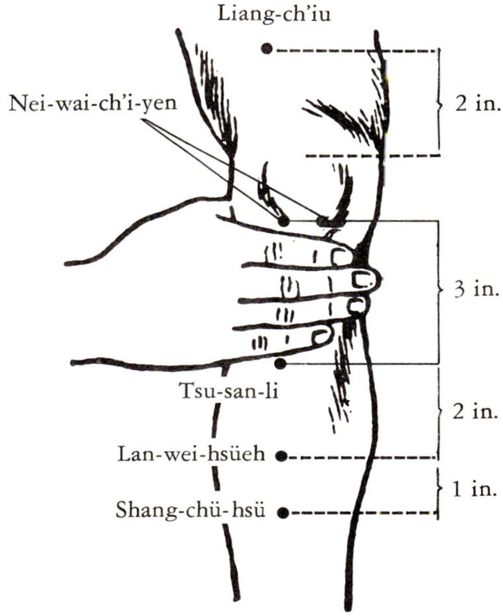

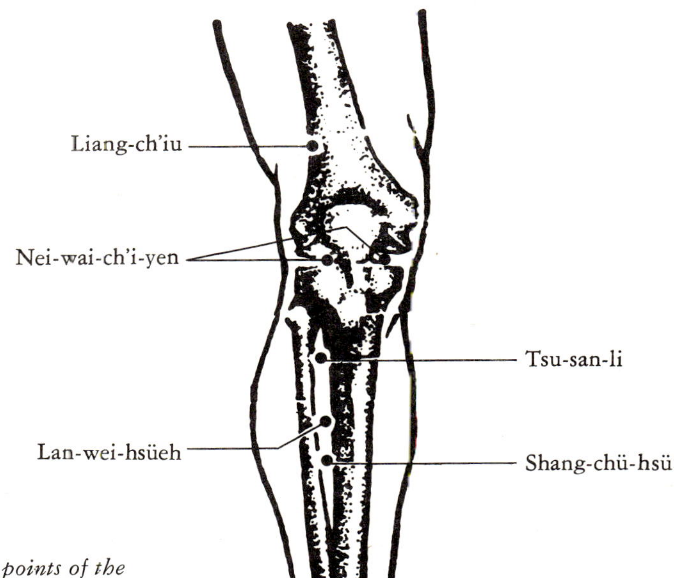

Fig. 34
Acupuncture points of the lower thigh and upper leg, anterior surface

11. Lan-wei-hsüeh, *pretibial #2 or appendix point (Fig. 34)*

Location. 2.0 inches directly distal to the point Tsu-san-li (LE–10). When appendicitis is present, point tenderness will be elicited when digital pressure is applied on the point.
Indications. Appendicitis.
Technique. Perpendicular insertion 1.5 to 2.0 inches deep.

12. Shang-chü-hsü, *pretibial #3 (Fig. 34)*

Location. 6.0 inches directly distal to the point where the lateral and apical (distal) margins of the patella intersect and 1.0 inches lateral to the tibia. It is also 1.0 inches distal to the point Lan-wei-hsüeh (LE–11).
Indications. Abdominal pain, diarrhea, and appendicitis.
Technique. Perpendicular insertion 1.0 to 2.0 inches deep.
Moxa heating. 5 to 20 minutes.

13. Chiai-ch'i, *dorsum of ankle (Fig. 35)*

Location. Directly in line with the second toe, in the groove between the tendons of the tibialis anterior and the extensor hallucis longus at the level of the center of the medial malleolus.
Indications. Painful disorders of the ankle, and paralysis of the lower extremity.
Technique. Perpendicular insertion, in the direction of the calcaneum, 0.5 to 1.0 inches deep.
Moxa heating. 5 to 10 minutes.

14. Nei-t'ing, *inter second and third metatarsals (Fig. 35)*

Location. On the dorsum of the foot between the second and third metatarsals and one index finger's width proximal to the corresponding metatarso-phalangeal joints.

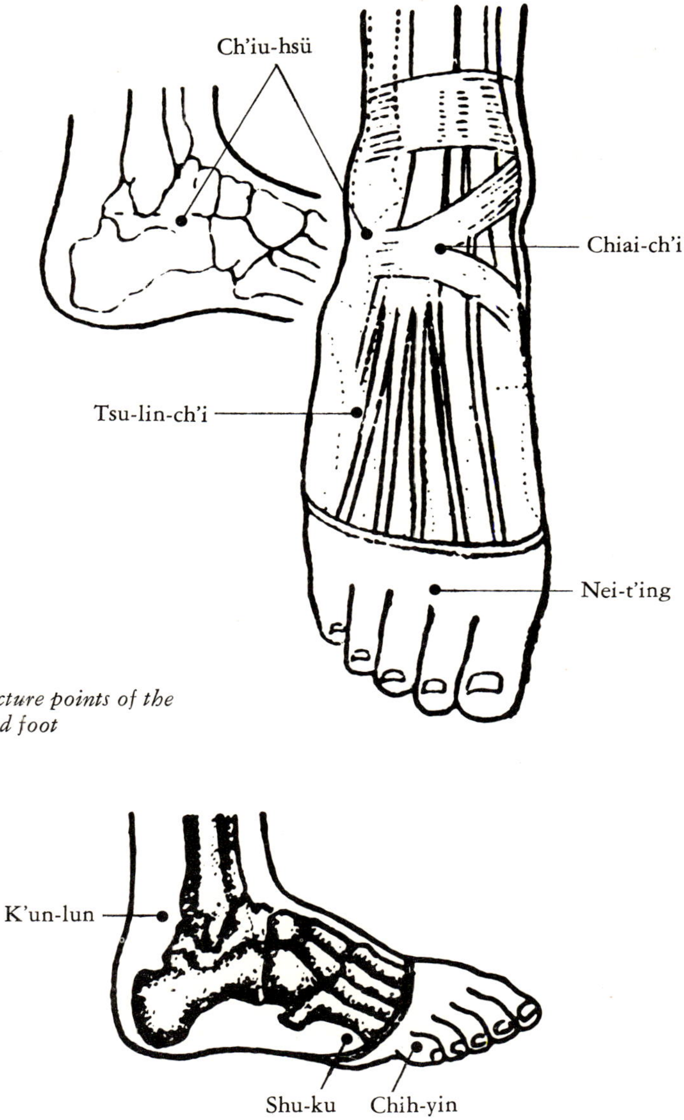

Fig. 35
Acupuncture points of the ankle and foot

Indications. Toothache, tonsillitis, tic douloureux, and headache.
Technique. Diagonal insertion towards the calcaneum to a depth of 0.2 to 0.5 inches.
Moxa heating. 5 to 10 minutes.

15. Yang-lin-ch'üan, *anterior to neck of fibula (Fig. 36)*

Location. Immediately anterior to the neck of the fibula.
Indications. Rib pain, diseases of the gallbladder and bile ducts, paralysis of the lower extremity, and painful disorders of the knee.
Technique. Perpendicular insertion to a depth of 0.5 to 2.0 inches.
Moxa heating. 5 to 15 minutes.

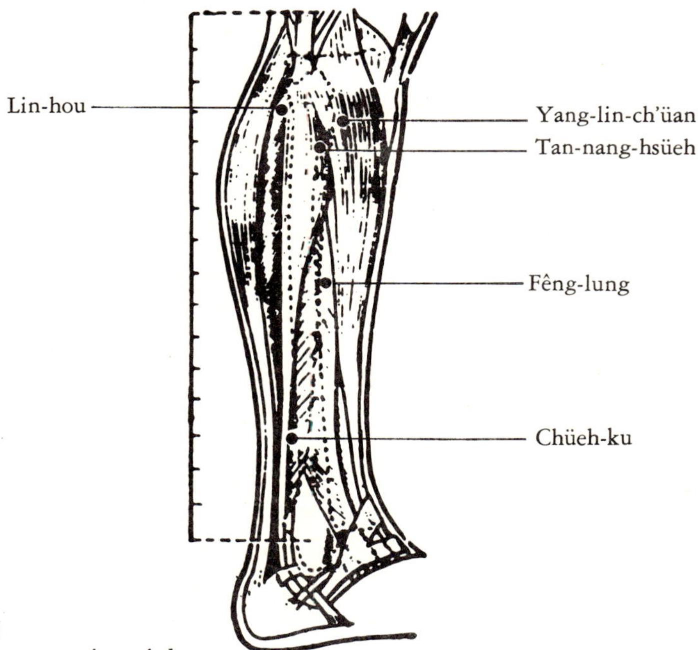

Fig. 36
Acupuncture points of the leg, lateral surface

16. Tan-nang-hsüeh, *proximal fibula or gallbladder point (Fig. 36)*

Location. Between 1.0 to 2.0 inches directly distal to the point for Yang-lin-ch'üan (LE–15). In a patient afflicted with pain from diseases of the gallbladder and bile ducts, point tenderness will be elicited upon applying digital pressure on the point.
Indications. Diseases of the gallbladder and bile ducts.
Technique. Perpendicular insertion to a depth of 1.0 to 2.0 inches.

17. Chüeh-ku, *distal fibula (Fig. 36)*

Location. 3.0 inches proximal to the lateral malleolus and between the fibula and the tendon of the peroneus longus.
Indications. Paralysis of the lower extremity, torticollis, and painful disorders of the ankle.
Technique. Perpendicular insertion 1.0 to 2.0 inches deep.
Moxa heating. 5 to 10 minutes.

18. Ch'iu-hsü, *lateral malleolus (Fig. 35)*

Location. At the point where the anterior and distal margins of the lateral malleolus intersect.
Indications. Painful disorders of the ankle, and rib pain.
Technique. Perpendicular insertion 1.0 to 1.5 inches deep.
Moxa heating. 5 to 10 minutes.

19. Tsu-lin-ch'i, *inter fourth and fifth metatarsals (Fig. 35)*

Location. On the dorsum of the foot between the fourth and fifth metatarsals and immediately lateral to the tendon of the extensor digitorum longus.
Indications. Suppression of lactation, mastitis, rib pain, headache, dizziness, and foot pain.
Technique. Perpendicular insertion 0.3 to 0.5 inches deep.
Moxa heating. 5 to 10 minutes.

20. Wei-chung, *popliteal fossa (Fig. 31)*

Location. At the center of the popliteal fossa.
Indications. Sciatica, lumbago, paralysis of the lower extremity,
Technique. Perpendicular insertion 0.5 to 1.0 inches deep. This is also a point for blood-letting.
Moxa heating. 3 to 5 minutes.

21. Ch'êng-san, *gastrocnemius (Fig. 31)*

Location. At the distal margin of the gastrocnemius muscle and between its medial and lateral heads. Hyperextension of the lower extremity will accentuate the outline of the muscle.
Indications. Sciatica, rectal prolapse, spasm of the gastrocnemius muscle, paralysis of the lower extremity, and pain of the sole of the foot.
Technique. Perpendicular insertion 1.0 to 2.5 inches deep.
Moxa heating. 5 to 15 minutes.

22. K'un-lun, *posterior to lateral malleolus (Fig. 35)*

Location. Midpoint between the posterior margin of the lateral malleolus and the Achilles tendon.
Indications. Paralysis of the lower extremity, sciatica, and painful disorders of the ankle.
Technique. Perpendicular insertion 0.5 inches deep.
Moxa heating. 5 to 15 minutes.

23. Shu-ku, *fifth metatarsal (Fig. 35)*

Location. Immediately beneath the fifth metatarsal and proximal to the fifth metatarso-phalangeal joint.
Indications. Headache, dizziness, and low back pain.
Technique. Perpendicular insertion 0.3 to 0.5 inches deep.
Moxa heating. 5 to 10 minutes.

24. Chih-yin, *base of fifth toenail (Fig. 35)*

Location. At the point where the lateral and proximal margins of the fifth toenail intersect.
Indications. Malposition of fetus and headache.
Technique. Diagonal insertion towards the base of the toe to a depth of 0.1 to 0.2 inches.
Moxa heating. 10 to 30 minutes.

25. Hsüeh-hai, *medial supra patella (Fig. 37)*

Location. At the center of the distal portion of the vastus medialis muscle, at a level 2.0 inches proximal to the patella. With the knee in 90° flexion, the practitioner, by cupping his hand over the patient's patella, can also locate the point immediately distal to the tip of his thumb.
Indications. Neurodermatitis, hives, pruritus, and menstrual irregularities.
Technique. Perpendicular insertion 1.0 to 2.0 inches deep.
Moxa heating. 5 to 15 minutes.

26. Yin-lin-ch'üan, *posterior proximal tibia (Fig. 37)*

Location. At the posterior edge of the tibia and immediately distal to its medial condyle. It is at the level of and opposite the point Yang-lin-ch'üan (LE–15).
Indications. Abdominal distention, diarrhea, menstrual irregularity, urinary retention, edema, and painful disorders of the knee.
Technique. Perpendicular insertion 1.0 to 3.0 inches deep.
Moxa heating. 5 to 15 minutes.

27. San-yin-chiao, *posterior to distal tibia (Fig. 38)*

Do not use this point in pregnant women.

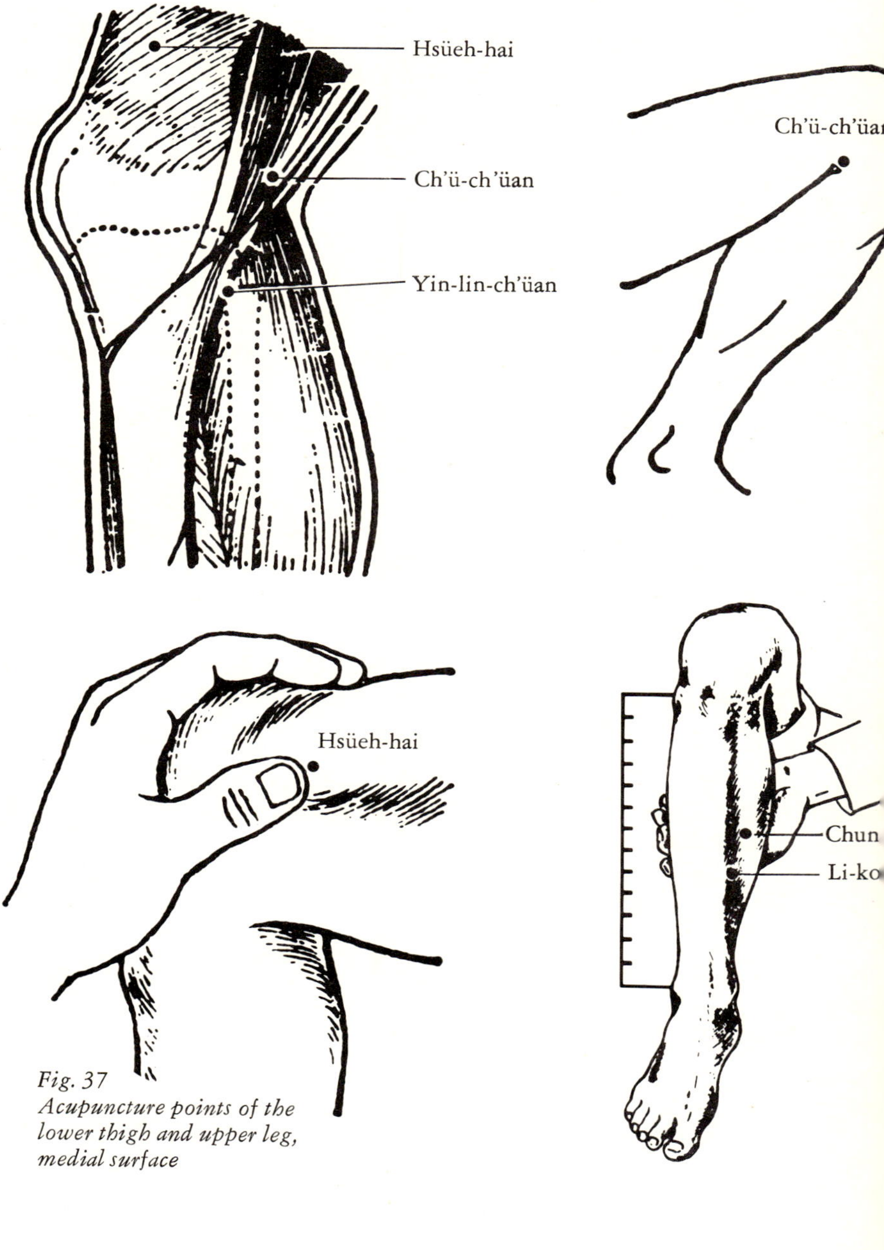

Fig. 37
Acupuncture points of the lower thigh and upper leg, medial surface

Location. 3.0 inches proximal to the medial malleolus and immediately posterior to the tibia.
Indications. Urological and gynecological disorders, neurasthenia, lower abdominal pain, diarrhea, insomnia, neurodermatitis, pruritus, and hives.
Technique. Perpendicular insertion 0.5 to 1.5 inches deep.
Moxa heating. 10 to 20 minutes.

28. Shang-ch'iu, *medial malleolus (Fig. 38)*

Location. At the point where the anterior and distal margins of the medial malleolus intersect.
Indications. Painful disorders of the ankle and indigestion.
Technique. Perpendicular insertion 0.3 to 0.5 inches deep.
Moxa heating. 5 to 20 minutes.

29. Kung-sun, *first metatarsal (Fig. 38)*

Location. Immediately beneath the first metatarsal and 1.0 inches proximal to the first metatarso-phalangeal joint.
Indications. Gastralgia, abdominal pain, and diarrhea.
Technique. Perpendicular insertion 0.7 to 1.0 inches deep.
Moxa heating. 5 to 15 minutes.

30. Yin-pê, *first toenail (Fig. 38)*

Location. At the intersection of the medial margin and the base of the first toenail.
Indications. Menorrhagia, uterine bleeding, and abdominal pain.
Technique. Diagonal insertion towards the base of the toe 0.1 to 0.2 inches deep.
Moxa heating. 5 to 20 minutes.

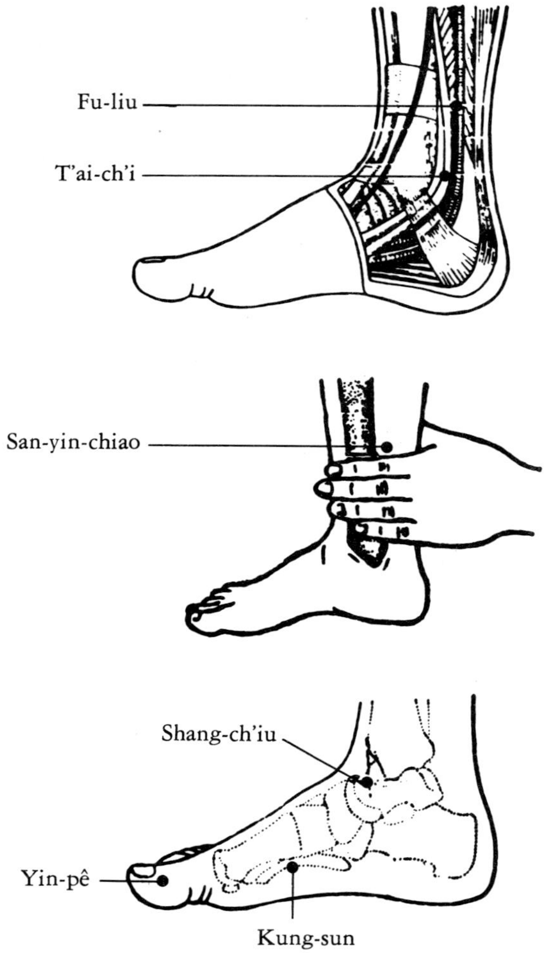

Fig. 38
Acupuncture points of the lower leg and foot, medial surface

31. Ch'ü-ch'üan, *medial popliteal fold (Fig. 37)*

Location. At the medial tip of the popliteal fold when the knee is flexed.
Indications. Nocturnal emission, dysuria, impotence, and painful disorders of the knee.
Technique. Perpendicular insertion 1.0 to 1.5 inches deep.
Moxa heating. 5 to 15 minutes.

32. Li-kou, *posterior to mid-tibia (Fig. 37)*

Location. 5.0 inches proximal to the medial malleolus and immediately posterior to the tibia.
Indications. Pelvic inflammatory diseases, renal failure, nocturnal emission, and impotence.
Technique. Perpendicular insertion 0.5 to 1.0 inches deep.
Moxa heating. 3 to 5 minutes.

33. T'ai-ch'ung, *inter first and second metatarsals (Fig. 39)*

Location. Between the first and second metatarsals and 2.0 inches proximal to the corresponding metatarso-phalangeal joints.
Indications. Headache, dizziness, hypertension, metrorrhagia, and mastitis.
Technique. Diagonal insertion towards the calcaneum 0.5 to 1.0 inches deep.
Moxa heating. 5 to 15 minutes.

34. T'ai-ch'i, *posterior to medial malleolus (Fig. 38)*

Location. On the medial surface of the ankle, at the midpoint of a line drawn from the posterior border of the medial malleolus to the Achilles tendon.
Indications. Low backache, hematuria, disorders of the reproduc-

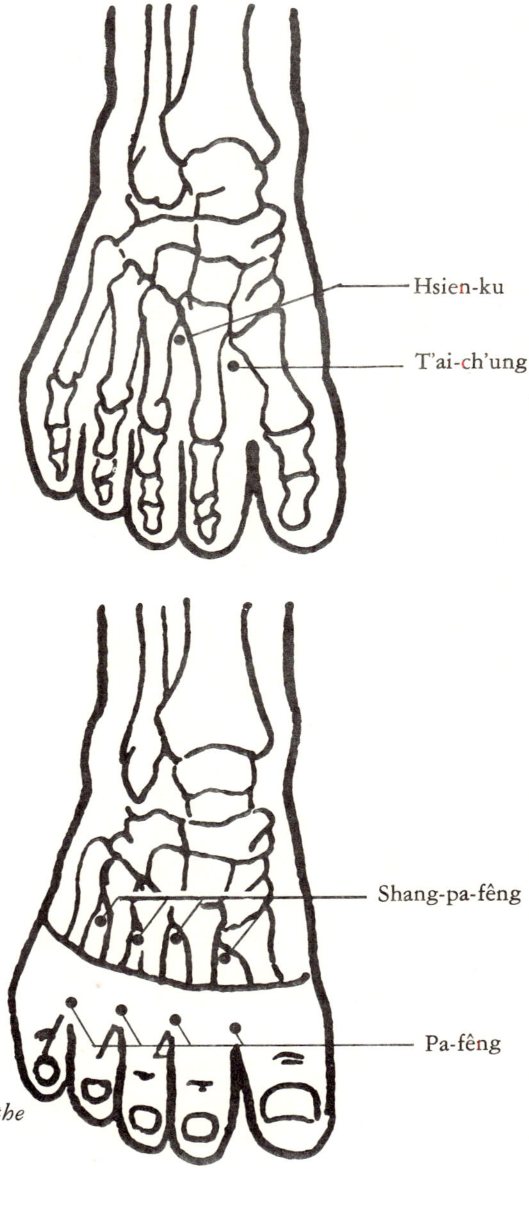

Fig. 39
Acupuncture points of the foot, dorsal surface

tive system, pain of the sole of the foot, paralysis of the lower extremity, and nervous breakdown.
Technique. Perpendicular insertion 0.3 to 0.5 inches deep.
Moxa heating. 5 to 15 minutes.

35. Fu-liu, *posterior to distal tibia (Fig. 38)*

Location. 2.0 inches directly proximal to the point T'ai-ch'i (LE–34).
Indications. Edema, excessive perspiration, and paralysis of the lower extremity.
Technique. Perpendicular insertion to a depth of 1.0 to 1.5 inches.
Moxa heating. 5 to 20 minutes.

36. Yung-ch'üan, *sole of foot (Fig. 40)*

Location. At the midline of the sole of the foot at a point one-third the distance of a line drawn from the third metatarso-phalangeal joint to the heel.
Indications. Headache, sun-stroke, and shock.
Technique. Perpendicular insertion 0.5 to 1.0 inches deep.
Moxa heating. 5 to 10 minutes.

37. Pa-fêng, *inter metatarso-phalangeal joints (Fig. 39)*

Location. 0.5 inches proximal to the web of the toes.
Indications. Pain, numbness, and inflammatory conditions of the dorsum of the foot and the toes.
Technique. Perpendicular insertion 0.5 inches deep.
Moxa heating. 5 to 10 minutes.

38. Shang-pa-fêng, *inter proximal metatarsals (Fig. 39)*

Location. Between the metatarsals and immediately distal to their bases.

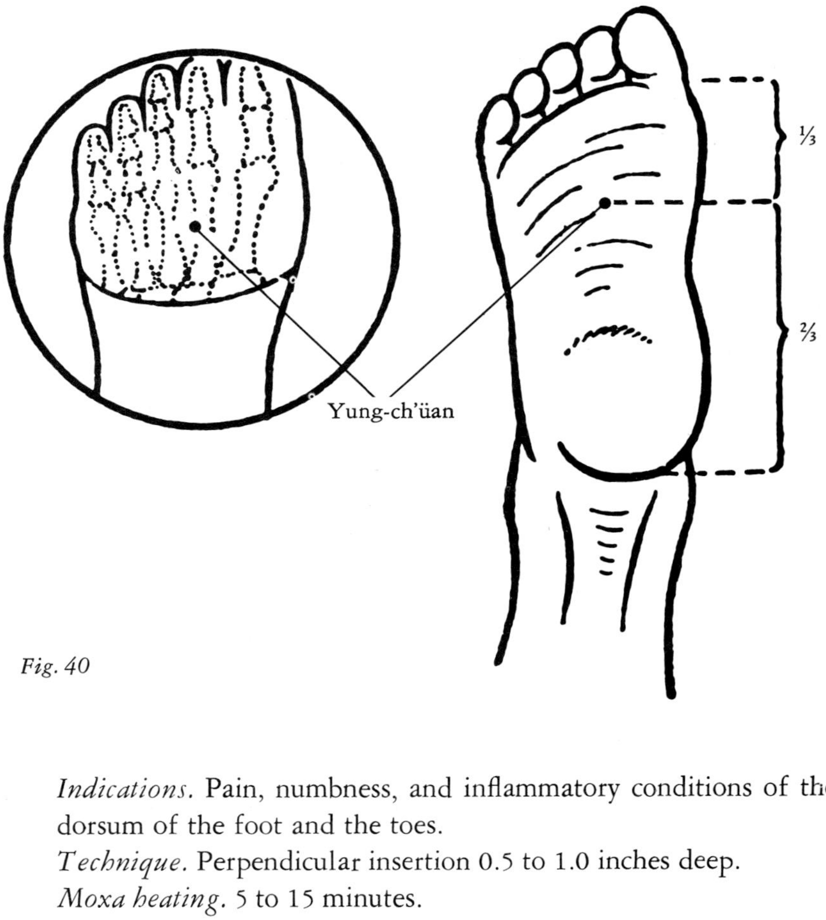

Fig. 40

Indications. Pain, numbness, and inflammatory conditions of the dorsum of the foot and the toes.
Technique. Perpendicular insertion 0.5 to 1.0 inches deep.
Moxa heating. 5 to 15 minutes.

39. Lin-hou, *posterior to neck of fibula (Fig. 36)*

Location. Immediately posterior to the neck of the fibula.
Indications. Sciatica and paralysis of the lower extremity.
Technique. Perpendicular insertion to a depth of 0.3 to 0.5 inches.
Moxa heating. 5 to 15 minutes.

40. Chung-tu *(Fig. 37)*

Location. 7.0 inches proximal to the medial malleolus and immediately posterior to the tibia.
Indications. Menorrhagia, pain of the leg, and colic.
Technique. Perpendicular insertion 0.5 to 1.5 inches deep.
Moxa heating. 3 to 5 minutes.

41. Fêng-lung *(Fig. 36)*

Location. 8.0 inches directly proximal to the anterior border of the lateral malleolus.
Indications. Cough, excessive phlegm, asthma, hemiplegia, headache, dizziness, and pharyngitis.
Technique. Perpendicular insertion 0.5 to 1.5 inches deep.
Moxa heating. 5 to 10 minutes.

42. Hsien-ku, *inter second and third metatarsals (Fig. 39)*

Location. Between the second and third metatarsals and immediately distal to their bases.
Indications. Edema, borborygmus, and pain and swelling of the dorsum of the foot.
Technique. Perpendicular insertion 0.5 to 1.0 inch deep.
Moxa heating. 5 to 15 minutes.

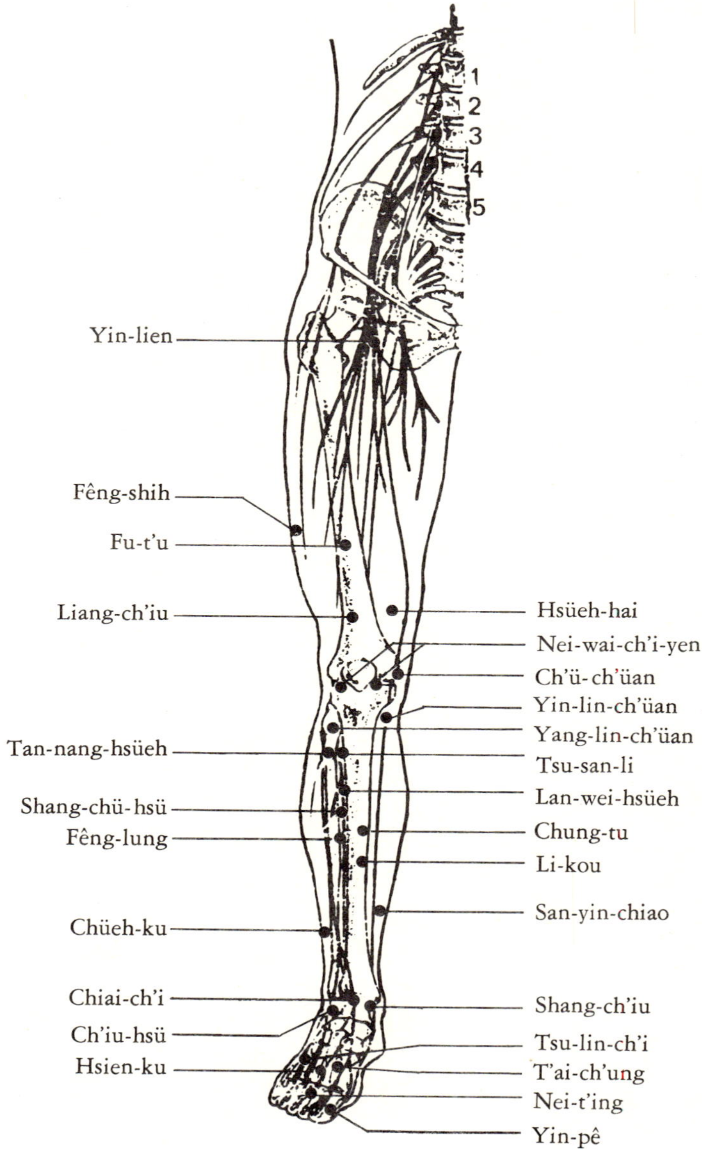

Fig. 41
Acupuncture points of the lower extremity, anterior surface

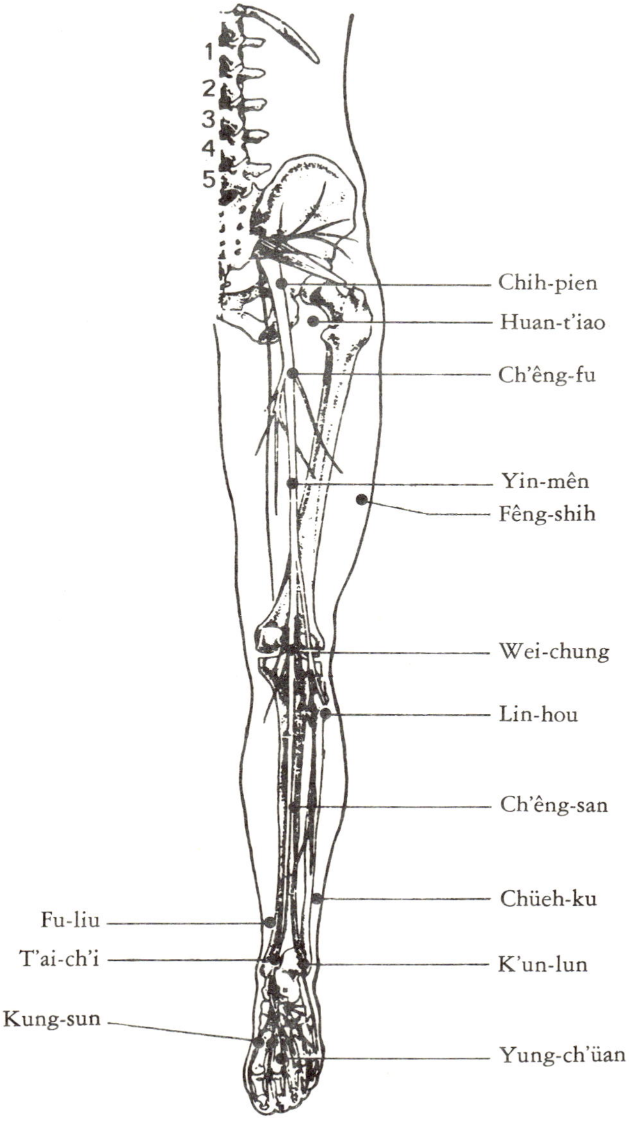

Fig. 42
Acupuncture points of the lower extremity, posterior surface

Table 3

SUMMARY OF ACUPUNCTURE POINTS OF LOWER EXTREMITY

LOCATION	NAME		COMMON INDICATIONS	SPECIFIC INDICATIONS
Hip	Huan-t'iao Chü-liao	Paralysis of the lower extremity, hip-joint pain	Painful disorders of the hip	Huan-t'iao: Sciatica, paralysis of the lower extremities
Thigh	Ch'êng-fu Yin-mên		Sciatica	Ch'êng-fu: Renal failure, acute Yin-mên: Lumbago
	Fêng-shih			Fêng-shih: Neurodermatitis of the thigh, lateral surface
	Yin-lien Fu-t'u		Disorders of the anterior surface of the thigh	Yin-lien: Painful disorders of the back and leg Fu-t'u: Painful disorders of the knee
Knee	Nei-wai-ch'i-yen			Painful disorders of the knee
Leg and Foot	Liang-ch'iu Tsu-san-li Lan-wei-hsüeh Shang-chü-hsü Chiai-ch'i Nei-t'ing	eases of the head local area, lysis of lower extremity	Diseases of the face, stomach, and intestines	Liang-ch'iu: Painful disorders of the knee Tsu-san-li: Hypertension, anemia, chronic fatigue Lan-wei-hsüeh: Appendicitis Shang-chü-hsü: Inflammation of the intestine Chiai-ch'i: Painful disorders of the

Tan-nang-hsueh Chüeh-ku Ch'iu-hsü Tsu-lin-ch'i Fêng-lung		the eye, ear, chest, and gallbladder	the knee Tan-nang-hsüeh: Diseases of the gall-bladder Chüeh-ku: Torticollis Ch'iu-hsü: Painful disorders of the ankle and rib cage Tsu-lin-ch'i: Painful disorders of the foot Fêng-lung: Cough, asthma
Wei-chung Ch'êng-san K'un-lun Shu-ku Chih-yin		Diseases of the neck, eye, and nose; lumbago, sciatica	Wei-chung: Lumbago, painful disorders of the knee Ch'êng-san: Gastrocnemius spasm K'un-lun: Painful disorders of the ankle Shu-ku: Headache, dizziness Chih-yin: Malposition of fetus
Hsüeh-hai Yin-lin-ch'üan San-yin-chiao Shang-ch'iu Kung-sun Yin-pê Chung-tu	Paralysis of lower extremity, diseases of abdomen and local area, urological disorders	Disease of the stomach, intestines, and abdomen	Hsüeh-hai: Pruritus, menstrual irregularities Yin-lin-ch'üan: Abdominal distention, edema, urinary retention, painful disorders of the knee San-yin-chiao: Pruritus, diarrhea, diseases of the reproductive system, insomnia Shang-ch'iu: Painful disorders of the ankle Kung-sun: Diseases of the stomach and intestines Yin-pê: Menstrual irregularity Chung-tu: Menorrhagia, colic, leg pain

Table 3 cont.

LOCATION	NAME	COMMON INDICATIONS		SPECIFIC INDICATIONS
Leg and Foot	Ch'ü-ch'üan Li-kou T'ai-ch'ung	Paralysis of lower extremity, diseases of abdomen and local area, urological disorders	Diseases of the liver	Ch'ü-ch'üan: Painful disorders of the knee and nocturnal emission Li-kou: Renal failure, impotence, nocturnal emission T'ai-ch'ung: Headache, dizziness, hypertension, mastitis, metrorrhagia
	Fu-liu T'ai-ch'i Yung-ch'üan		Diseases of the kidney	Fu-liu: Excessive perspiration, edema T'ai-ch'i: Painful disorders of the back and sole of foot Yung-ch'üan: Headache
Others	Pa-fêng Shang-pa-fêng Lin-hou Hsien-ku			Pa-fêng and Shang-pa-fêng: Painful disorders of the foot and toes Lin-hou: Sciatica, paralysis of lower extremities Hsien-ku: Edema, pain of foot

POINTS OF THE CHEST AND ABDOMEN

1. T'ien-t'u, *supra sternal notch (Figs. 43 and 44)*

Location. With the neck hyperextended, the point is located 0.5 inches superior to the sternal notch of the sternum.
Indications. Asthma, upper respiratory infections, pharyngitis, and diaphragmodynia.
Technique. Horizontal insertion, caudad behind the sternum, to a depth of 0.5 to 0.7 inches.
Moxa heating. 5 to 15 minutes.

2. Hsüan-chi, *manubrium sterni (Figs. 43 and 44)*

Location. 1.0 inches directly inferior to the point T'ien-t'u (CA–1).
Indications. Asthma.
Technique. Horizontal insertion, caudad, 0.5 to 1.0 inches deep.
Moxa heating. 5 to 15 minutes.

3. Tan-chung, *xiphi-sternal junction (Figs. 43 and 44)*

Location. At the xiphi-sternal junction, midpoint between the nipples.
Indications. Asthma, upper respiratory infections, and insufficiency of lactation.
Technique. Horizontal insertion, cephalad, 0.5 to 1.0 inches deep.
Moxa heating. 5 to 15 minutes.

4. Ru-kêng, *nipple line (Fig. 43)*

Location. Between the fifth and sixth ribs directly inferior to the nipple.
Indications. Mastitis and insufficiency of lactation.
Technique. Horizontal insertion in a cephalad, medial, or lateral direction to a depth of 0.5 to 1.5 inches.
Moxa heating. 5 to 20 minutes.

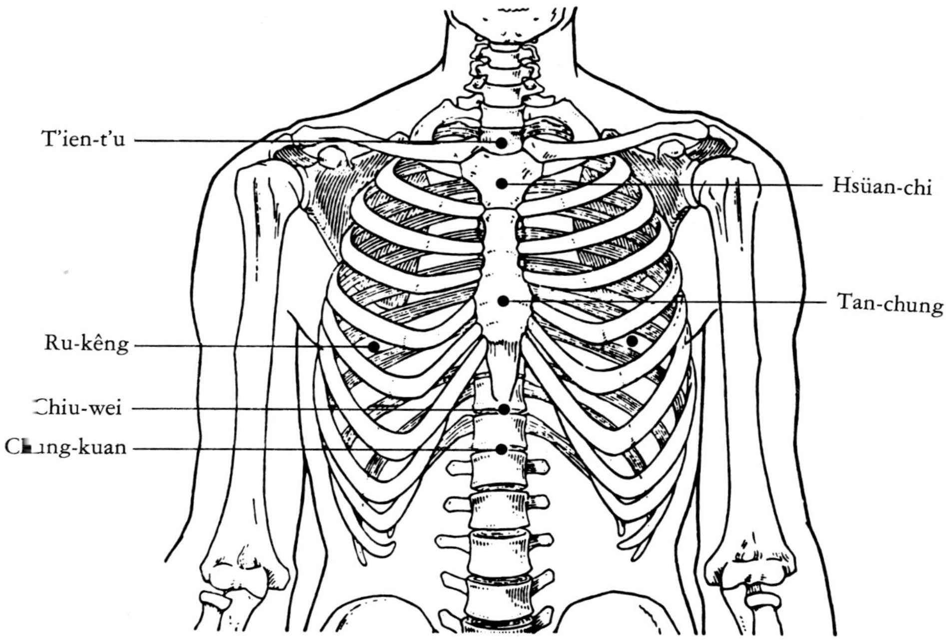

Fig. 43
Acupuncture points of the chest

5. Chiu-wei, *xiphoid process (Figs. 43 and 44)*

Location. 0.5 inches inferior to the xiphoid process.
Indications. Psychoses, epilepsy, angina pectoris, emesis, and gastralgia.
Technique. Diagonal insertion (30° angle), caudad, 1.5 to 2.0 inches deep.
Moxa heating. 5 to 15 minutes.

6. Chung-kuan, *epigastrium (Figs. 43 and 44)*

Location. At the epigastrium, 3.0 inches directly inferior to Chiu-wei (CA–5).
Indications. Gastralgia, emesis, nausea, indigestion, gastroptosis, and abdominal distention.
Technique. Perpendicular insertion 1.0 to 2.0 inches deep.
Moxa heating. 10 to 20 minutes.

7. Ch'i-chung, *umbilicus (Fig. 44)*

Location. At the umbilicus.
Indications. Abdominal pain and diarrhea.
Technique. No needle insertion is recommended.
Moxa heating. 20 to 30 minutes.

8. Ch'i-hai, *upper hypogastrium (Fig. 44)*

Do not use this point in pregnant women.
Location. 1.5 inches directly inferior to the umbilicus.
Indications. Nocturnal emission, impotence, menstrual cramps, menstrual irregularity, urinary retention, enuresis, diarrhea, and abdominal distention.
Technique. Diagonal insertion, caudad, 0.8 to 2.0 inches deep. The bladder should be emptied before needle insertion.
Moxa heating. 20 to 30 minutes.

9. Kuan-yüan, *mid-hypogastrium (Fig. 44)*

Do not use this point in pregnant women.
Location. 3.0 inches directly inferior to the umbilicus.
Indications. Nocturnal emission, impotence, menstrual cramps, menstrual irregularity, urinary retention, enuresis, diarrhea, and abdominal distention.
Technique. Diagonal insertion, caudad, 0.8 to 2.0 inches deep. The

bladder should be emptied before needle insertion.
Moxa heating. 20 to 30 minutes.

10. Chung-chi, *lower hypogastrium (Fig. 44)*

Do not use this point in pregnant women.
Location. 4.0 inches directly inferior to the umbilicus.
Indications. Nocturnal emission, impotence, menstrual irregularity, excessive vaginal discharge, pelvic inflammatory disease, enuresis, urinary incontinence, and urinary retention.
Technique. Diagonal insertion, caudad, 0.8 to 2.0 inches deep. The bladder should be emptied before needle insertion.
Moxa heating. 20 to 30 minutes.

11. Ch'ü-ku, *symphysis pubis (Fig. 44)*

Location. Immediately superior to the symphysis pubis.
Indications. Nocturnal emission, impotence, menstrual irregular-

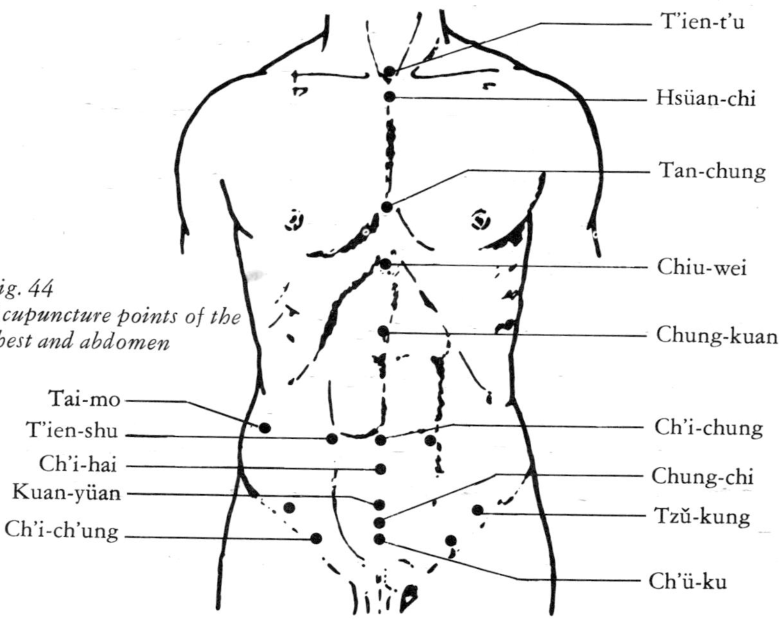

Fig. 44
Acupuncture points of the chest and abdomen

ity, excessive vaginal discharge, pelvic inflammatory disease, enuresis, urinary incontinence, and urinary retention.
Technique. Diagonal insertion, caudad, 0.8 to 2.0 inches deep. The bladder should be emptied prior to needle insertion.
Moxa heating. 20 to 30 minutes.

12. T'ien-shu, *paraumbilical (Fig. 44)*

Location. 2.0 inches lateral to the umbilicus.
Indications. Abdominal distention, diarrhea, menstrual disorders, constipation, and intestinal spasm.
Technique. Perpendicular insertion 0.7 to 1.2 inches deep.
Moxa heating. 10 to 20 minutes.

13. Ch'i-ch'ung, *lower inguinal (Fig. 44)*

Location. 2.0 inches lateral to the point Ch'ü-ku (CA–11).
Indications. Disorders of the male and female reproductive organs.
Technique. Perpendicular insertion 0.5 to 1.0 inches deep.
Moxa heating. 5 to 15 minutes.

14. Tzŭ-kung, *upper inguinal or uterus point (Fig. 44)*

Location. 3.0 inches lateral to the point Chung-chi (CA–10).
Indications. Gynecological disorders.
Technique. Perpendicular insertion 1.5 to 2.0 inches deep.
Moxa heating. 10 to 20 minutes.

15. Tai-mo, *flank (Fig. 44)*

Location. Directly below the tip of the eleventh rib and at the level of the umbilicus.
Indications. Menstrual irregularities and cramps, endometritis, and hernia pain.
Technique. Perpendicular insertion 0.5 to 1.0 inch deep.
Moxa heating. 3 to 7 minutes.

Table 4

SUMMARY OF ACUPUNCTURE POINTS OF THE CHEST AND ABDOMEN

LOCATION	NAME	COMMON INDICATIONS	SPECIFIC INDICATIONS
Chest	T'ien-t'u Tan-chung Hsüan-chi Ru-kêng	Diseases of the chest, including diseases of the upper respiratory system	T'ien-t'u: Diseases of the throat Tan-chung, Ru-kêng: Diseases of the breast
Upper Abdomen	Chiu-wei Chung-kuan	Diseases of upper abdomen, mainly diseases of the stomach	Chiu-wei: Mental disorders, epilepsy, chest pain Chung-kuan: Stomach and intestinal disorders
Lower Abdomen	Ch'i-chung T'ien-shu Tai-mo	Intestinal disorders	T'ien-shu: Menstrual disorders Tai-mo: Menstrual disorders, hernia pain
	Ch'i-hai Kuan-yüan Chung-chi Ch'ü-ku	Urinary tract disorders and disorders of the reproductive system	Ch'i-hai, Kuan-yüan: Intestinal disorders
	Ch'i-ch'ung Tsŭ-kung	Disorders of the reproductive system	Tsŭ-kung: Gynecological disorders

POINTS OF THE BACK

1. Ta-ch'ui, *C7–T1 (Fig.45)*

Location. In the midline between the seventh cervical vertebra (C7) and the first thoracic vertebra (T1).
Indications. Fever, malaria, schizophrenia, epilepsy, and asthma.
Technique. Perpendicular insertion 0.5 to 0.8 inches deep.
Moxa heating. 5 to 20 minutes.

2. T'ao-tao, *T1–T2 (Fig. 45)*

Location. In the midline between the first and second thoracic vertebrae.
Indications. Fever, malaria, and schizophrenia.
Technique. Perpendicular insertion to a depth of 0.5 to 0.8 inches.
Moxa heating. 5 to 20 minutes.

3. Ch'uan-hsi, *paravertebral C7 (Fig. 45)*

Location. 0.5 inches lateral to the seventh cervical vertebra.
Indications. Torticollis, asthma, and cough.
Technique. Perpendicular insertion 0.5 to 1.0 inches deep.
Moxa heating. 5 to 15 minutes.

4. Fêng-mên, *paravertebral T2–T3 (Fig. 45)*

Location. 1.5 inches lateral to the midline and at a level between the second and third thoracic vertebrae.
Indications. Influenza, pneumonia, bronchitis, asthma, pleurisy, pertussis, and upper backache.
Technique. Diagonal insertion, caudad, 0.3 to 0.5 inches deep.
Moxa heating. 5 to 15 minutes.

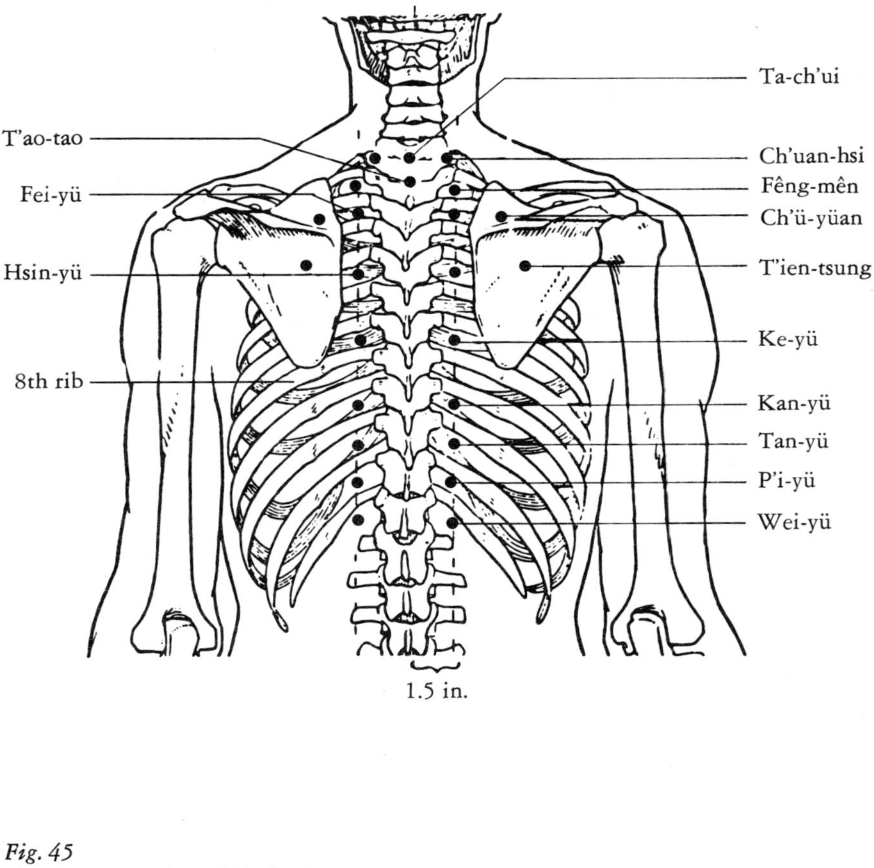

Fig. 45
Acupuncture points of the back

5. Fei-yü, *paravertebral T3–T4 or lung point (Fig. 45)*

Location. 1.5 inches lateral to the midline and at a level between the third and fourth thoracic vertebrae.
Indications. Pneumonia, upper respiratory infections, asthma, pulmonary tuberculosis, pleurisy, cough, and upper backache.
Technique. Diagonal insertion, caudad, 0.3 to 0.5 inches deep.
Moxa heating. 5 to 15 minutes.

6. Hsin-yü, *paravertebral T5–T6 or heart point (Fig. 45)*

Location. 1.5 inches lateral to the midline and at a level between the fifth and sixth thoracic vertebrae.
Indications. Nervous breakdown, insomnia, palpitations, and schizophrenia.
Technique. Diagonal insertion, caudad, 0.3 to 0.5 inches deep.
Moxa heating. 5 to 15 minutes.

7. Ke-yü, *paravertebral T7–T8 or diaphragm point (Fig. 45)*

Location. 1.5 inches lateral to the midline and at a level between the seventh and eighth thoracic vertebrae.
Indications. Diaphragmodynia, upper backache, cough, asthma, and anemia.
Technique. Diagonal insertion, caudad, 0.3 to 0.5 inches deep.
Moxa heating. 5 to 15 minutes.

8. Ch'ü-yüan, *supraspinous fossa of scapula (Fig. 45)*

Location. Immediately superior to the medial border of the spine of the scapula in the supraspinous fossa.
Indications. Painful disorders of the scapula and shoulder.
Technique. Perpendicular insertion to a depth of 0.5 to 0.8 inches.
Moxa heating. 5 to 15 minutes.

9. T'ien-tsung, *infraspinous fossa of scapula (Fig. 45)*

Location. In the infraspinous fossa of the scapula at a point one-third the distance from the spine of the scapula to its inferior angle and midway between its medial and lateral borders.
Indications. Painful disorders of the shoulder, upper arm, and scapula.
Technique. Perpendicular insertion 0.5 to 1.5 inches deep.
Moxa heating. 5 to 15 minutes.

10. Kan-yü, *paravertebral T9–T10 or liver point (Fig. 45)*

Location. 1.5 inches lateral to the midline and at a level between the ninth and tenth thoracic vertebrae.
Indications. Hepatitis, backache, and diseases of the eye.
Technique. Diagonal insertion, caudad, 0.3 to 0.5 inches deep.
Moxa heating. 5 to 15 minutes.

11. Tan-yü, *paravertebral T10–T11 or gallbladder point (Fig. 45)*

Location. 1.5 inches lateral to the midline and at a level between the tenth and eleventh thoracic vertebrae.
Indications. Diseases of the gallbladder and bile ducts, hepatitis, and backache.
Technique. Diagonal insertion, caudad, to a depth of 0.3 to 0.5 inches.
Moxa heating. 5 to 15 minutes.

12. P'i-yü, *paravertebral T11–T12 or spleen point (Fig. 46)*

Location. 1.5 inches lateral to the midline and at a level between the eleventh and twelfth thoracic vertebrae.
Indications. Gastralgia, indigestion, anemia, and backache.
Technique. Diagonal insertion, caudad, 0.3 to 0.5 inches deep.
Moxa heating. 5 to 20 minutes.

13. Wei-yü, *paravertebral T12–L1 or stomach point (Figs. 45 and 46)*

Location. 1.5 inches lateral to the midline and at a level between the twelfth thoracic and the first lumbar vertebrae.
Indications. Gastralgia, indigestion, anorexia, and backache.
Technique. Diagonal insertion, caudad, 0.3 to 0.5 inches deep.
Moxa heating. 5 to 20 minutes.

14. Ming-mên, *L2–L3 (Fig. 46)*

Location. In the midline, between the second and third lumbar vertebrae.
Indications. Lumbar disorders, nocturnal emission, and impotence.
Technique. Perpendicular insertion 0.5 to 0.8 inches deep. The needle should be directed slightly cephalad.
Moxa heating. 5 to 20 minutes.

15. Shêng-yü, *paravertebral L2–L3 or kidney point (Fig. 46)*

Location. 1.5 inches lateral to the midline and at a level between the second and third lumbar vertebrae.
Indications. Lumbar disorders, renal infections, renal colic, nocturnal emission, impotence, menstrual disorders, and nervous breakdown.
Technique. Perpendicular insertion 0.5 to 1.2 inches deep.
Moxa heating. 5 to 20 minutes.

16. Chih-shih, *paravertebral L2–L3 (Fig. 46)*

Location. 3.0 inches lateral to the midline and at a level between the second and third lumbar vertebrae.
Indications. Lumbar disorders, renal infections, renal colic, nocturnal emission, and diseases of the reproductive system.
Technique. Either perpendicular insertion 0.3 to 0.5 inches deep

or horizontal insertion, cephalad or caudad, 1.0 to 2.0 inches deep.
Moxa heating. 5 to 20 minutes.

17. Yao-yang-kuan, *L4–L5 (Fig. 46)*

Location. In the midline, between the fourth and fifth lumbar vertebrae.
Indications. Lumbar backache.
Technique. Perpendicular insertion 0.5 to 1.2 inches deep.
Moxa heating. 5 to 20 minutes.

18. Ta-ch'ang-yü, *paravertebral L4–L5 or large intestine point (Fig. 46)*

Location. 1.5 inches lateral to the midline and at a level between the fourth and fifth lumbar vertebrae.
Indications. Lumbar and sacro-iliac strain, sciatica, painful disorders of the hip, and intestinal ailments.
Technique. Perpendicular insertion 0.7 to 1.3 inches deep.
Moxa heating. 5 to 20 minutes.

19. Shih-ch'i-ch'ui-hsia, *L5–S1 (Fig. 46)*

Location. In the midline between the fifth lumbar and first sacral vertebrae.
Indications. Sacro-iliac and hip pain.
Technique. Perpendicular insertion 1.0 to 2.5 inches deep.
Moxa heating. 5 to 20 minutes.

20. Shang-liao, *first sacral foramen (Fig. 46)*

Do not use this point in pregnant women.
Location. At the first sacral foramen, that is, 1.0 inches lateral to the midline of the sacrum and at a level between the first and second sacral vertebrae.

Indications. Urinary problems, menstrual irregularity, induction of labor, reproductive disorders, low backache, and sciatica.
Technique. Perpendicular insertion 1.0 to 2.0 inches deep.
Moxa heating. 5 to 20 minutes.

21. Ts'ŭ-liao, *second sacral foramen (Fig. 46)*

Do not use this point in pregnant women.
Location. At the second sacral foramen.
Indications. Similar to the indications for Shang-liao (B–20).
Technique. Same as technique for Shang-liao (B–20).
Moxa heating. 5 to 20 minutes.

22. Hsiao-ch'ang-yü, *paravertebral S1–S2 or small intestine point (Fig. 46)*

Location. 1.5 inches lateral to the midline and at a level between the first and second sacral vertebrae.
Indications. Low backache, hip pain, and intestinal disorders.
Technique. Perpendicular insertion 0.5 to 1.5 inches deep.
Moxa heating. 5 to 20 minutes.

23. P'ang-k'uang-yü, *paravertebral S2–S3 or bladder point (Fig. 46)*

Location. 1.5 inches lateral to the midline and at a level between the second and third sacral vertebrae.
Indications. Urinary disorders and low backache.
Technique. Perpendicular insertion 0.5 to 1.5 inches deep.
Moxa heating. 5 to 20 minutes.

24. Chih-pien, *paravertebral S4–S5 (Fig. 46)*

Location. 3.0 inches lateral to the midline and at a level between the fourth and fifth sacral vertebrae.
Indications. Sciatica, paralysis of lower extremity, gluteal pain,

anal disorders, and hemorrhoids.
Technique. Perpendicular insertion 1.0 to 2.0 inches deep.
Moxa heating. 5 to 20 minutes.

25. Ch'ang-ch'iang, *anal (Fig. 46)*

Location. In the midline, midpoint between the apex or tip of the coccyx and the anus.
Indications. Hemorrhoids and rectal prolapse.
Technique. With the patient bent over, perpendicular insertion, cephalad between the rectum and the coccyx, to a depth of 0.5 to 1.0 inches.
Moxa heating. 5 to 20 minutes.

26. Chiai-ch'uan, *paravertebral S1, S2, S3 (Fig. 46)*

Location. 2.0 inches lateral to the midline and at the levels of the first, second, and third sacral vertebrae, a total of three points on each side.
Indications. Cough and asthma.
Technique. Perpendicular insertion to a depth of 1.0 to 1.5 inches.

27. Ch'i-hai-yü, *paravertebral L3–L4 (Fig. 46)*

Location. 1.5 inches lateral to the midline and at a level between the third and fourth lumbar vertebrae.
Indications. Lumbar pain.
Technique. Perpendicular insertion 0.5 to 1.5 inches deep.
Moxa heating. 5 to 15 minutes.

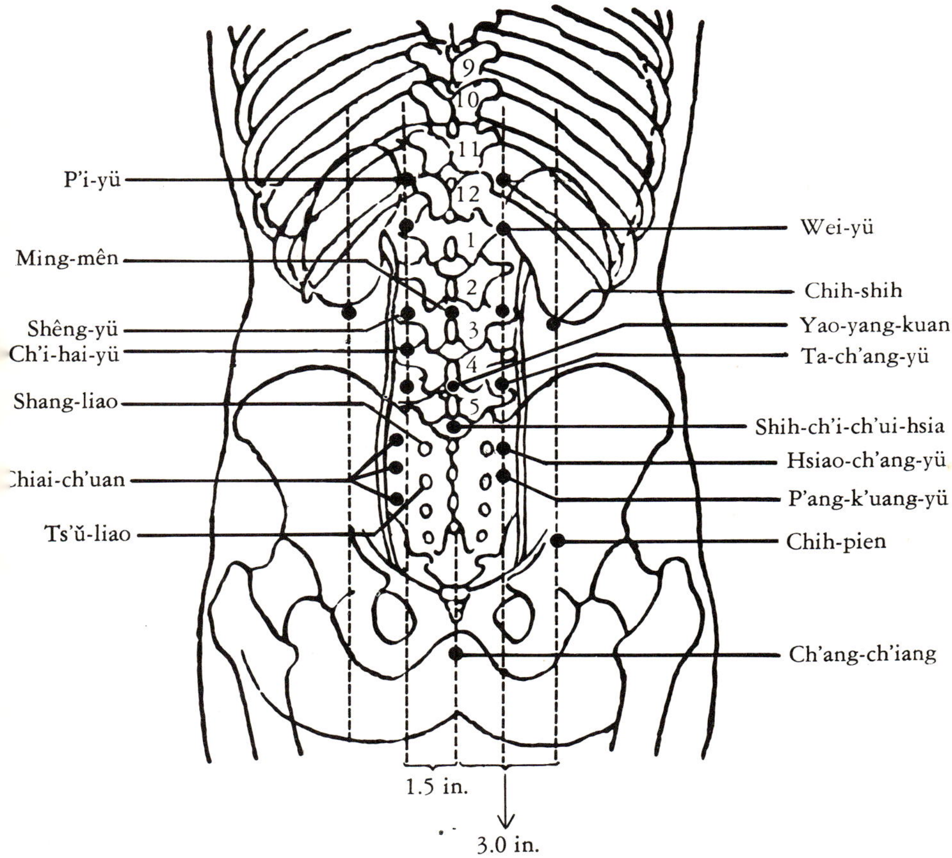

Fig. 46
Acupuncture points of the lower back

Table 5

SUMMARY OF ACUPUNCTURE POINTS OF THE BACK

LOCATION	NAME		COMMON INDICATIONS	SPECIFIC INDICATIONS
Cervico-Thoracic	Ta-ch'ui T'ao-tao	Diseases of heart and lung	Painful disorders of the vertebrae	Ta-ch'ui: Schizophrenia, asthma, fever, malaria T'ao-tao: Schizophrenia, fever, malaria
	Fêng-mên Fei-yü Ch'uan-hsi Hsin-yü Ke-yü		Local painful disorders	Fêng-mên: Influenza Fei-yü: Diseases of the lung Hsin-yü: Diseases of the heart, mental disorders Ke-yü: Anemia, spasm of diaphragm Ch'uan-hsi: Asthma
Thoraco-Lumbar	Kan-yü Tan-yü P'i-yü Wei-yü		Diseases of the liver, gall-bladder, spleen, stomach, and local soft tissue	Kan-yü: Diseases of the eye and liver Tan-yü: Diseases of the gallbladder P'i-yü and Wei-yü: Indigestion, gastralgia
Lumbo-Sacral	Ming-mên Yao-yang-kuan Shih-ch'i-ch'ui-hsia Ch'i-hai-yü		Diseases of the vertebrae	Ming-mên: Diseases of the male reproductive organ

	Shêng-yü Chih-shih Ta-ch'ang-yü Hsiao-ch'ang-yü P'ang-k'uang-yü Shang-liao Ts'ŭ-liao Chih-pien	Diseases of the kidney, intestines, urinary tract, and reproductive organs	Diseases of the local soft tissue	Shêng-yü, Chih-shih: Diseases of the urinary tract and reproductive organs Shang-liao, Ts'ŭ-liao: Diseases of the urinary tract and reproductive organs, sciatica Ta-ch'ang-yü, Hsiao-ch'ang-yü: Diseases of the intestines P'ang-k'uang-yü: Diseases of the urinary tract Chih-pien: Sciatica, paralysis of the lower extremity
Scapula	T'ien-tsung Ch'ü-yüan		Painful disorders of the shoulder	
Sacral	Chiai-ch'uan			Chiai-ch'uan: Cough, asthma
Anal	Ch'ang-ch'iang			Ch'ang-ch'iang: Hemorrhoids, rectal prolapse

POINTS OF THE EXTERNAL EAR

Acupuncture points of the external ear or auricle are, to a degree, unusual and unique in that all acupuncture points necessary for treatment of diseases of the entire body can be located in this one small organ. These points are noteworthy for achieving rapid alleviation of pain and are frequently and effectively utilized in acupuncture-anesthesia.

LOCATION OF ACUPUNCTURE POINTS OF THE EAR (SEE FIG. 48)

The auricle is pictured as a fetus in an inverted position in the uterus (see Fig. 47). With this in mind, it is possible to ascribe to each organ of the human body a corresponding area in the external ear in which is located the acupuncture point utilized for treatment of ailments as well as for inducing surgical analgesia for that particular organ. Thus,

1. The lobule of the auricle, or earlobe, contains acupuncture points for the eyes, the tongue, the teeth, the tonsils, the internal ear, and the jaws.
2. The antitragus is the location of ear points for the brain, the brain stem, the occiput, and the forehead. The subcortex, testis, ovary, and P'ing-ch'uan points are also located there.
3. The antihelix contains points for the toe, the ankle, the knee, the sciatic nerve, the buttocks, the abdomen, the chest, the neck, the coccyx, and the cervical, thoracic, and lumbosacral vertebrae.
4. The superior crus antihelicis contains the ear points for the lower extremities including the toes, the heel, the ankle, and the knee.
5. The inferior crus antihelicis is the location of points for the buttocks, the sciatic nerve, and the Chiao-kan (sympathetic nerve) point.
6. The triangular fossa contains points for the uterus, the hip joint, and the Shên-mên point.

7. The scaphoid fossa is the location of points for the upper extremities including the clavicle, the shoulder joint, the shoulder, the elbow, the wrist, and the fingers.
8. The tragus contains points for the nose, the throat, and the adrenal glands.
9. The incisura intertragica contains points for the endocrine, or hormonal system, and the scrotum.
10. The inferior concha is the location of points for the thorax, the thoracic contents including the heart, the lungs, the cardiac orifice, the esophagus, and the trachea. It also contains the San-chiao and the stomach points.
11. The superior concha contains points for the urinary bladder, the kidneys, the gallbladder, the pancreas, the liver, the spleen, the large and small intestines, and the appendix.
12. The crus helicis contains the point for the diaphragm.
13. The helix is the location of points for the rectum, the urethra, the external genitalia, and the ear apex.
14. The back of the ear contains points for the back of the body as well as a point for lowering blood pressure.

Selection of Acupuncture Points of the External Ear

As described in the preceding paragraph, each organ or structure of the body has a specific site on the auricle in which are located acupuncture points for treatment of its diseases or of symptoms arising from it. In addition, in accordance with medical theories, diseases of one organ may be due to afflictions of another organ. In such cases, the points for both organs are utilized. For example, practitioners of traditional Chinese medicine believe that diseases of the eye are related to disorders of the liver; therefore, acupuncture points specific for both organs are simultaneously used for treatment of these eye diseases. Furthermore, menstrual cramps are best treated by simultaneous stimulation of acupuncture points for the uterus as well as the

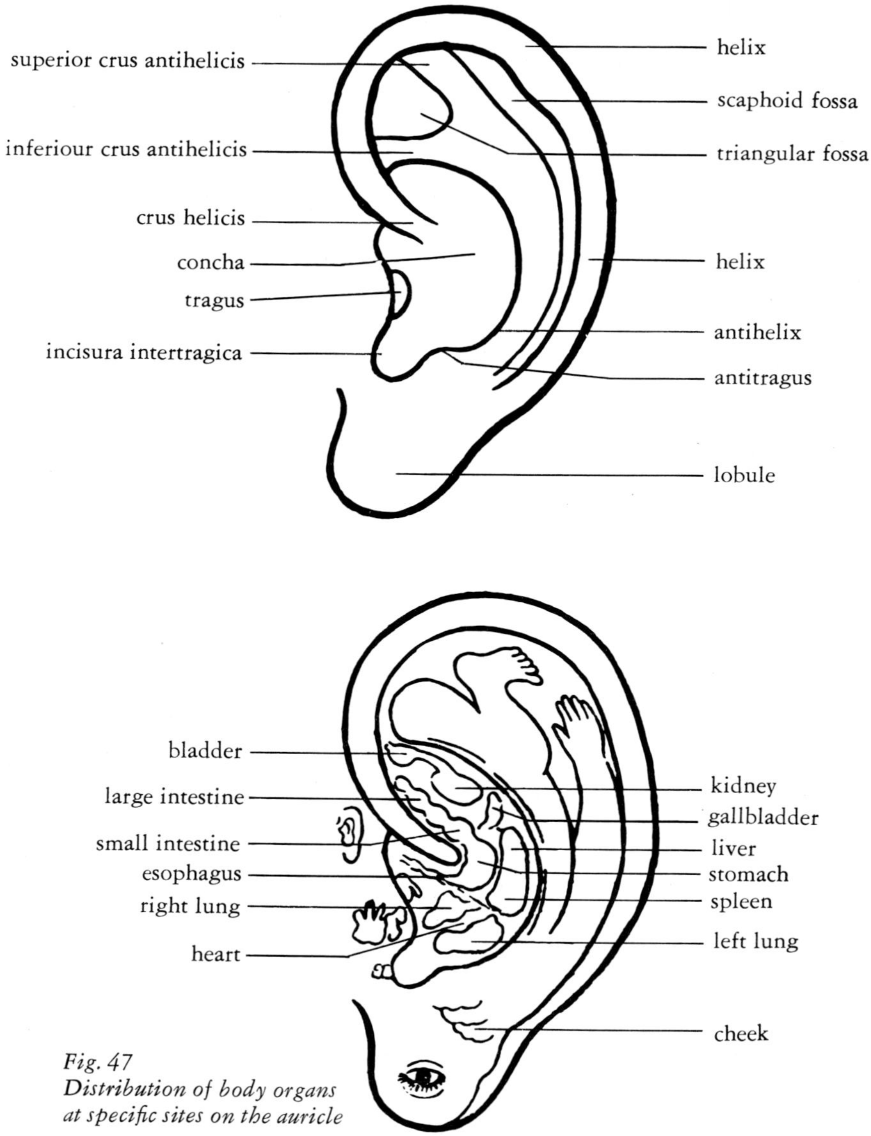

Fig. 47
Distribution of body organs at specific sites on the auricle

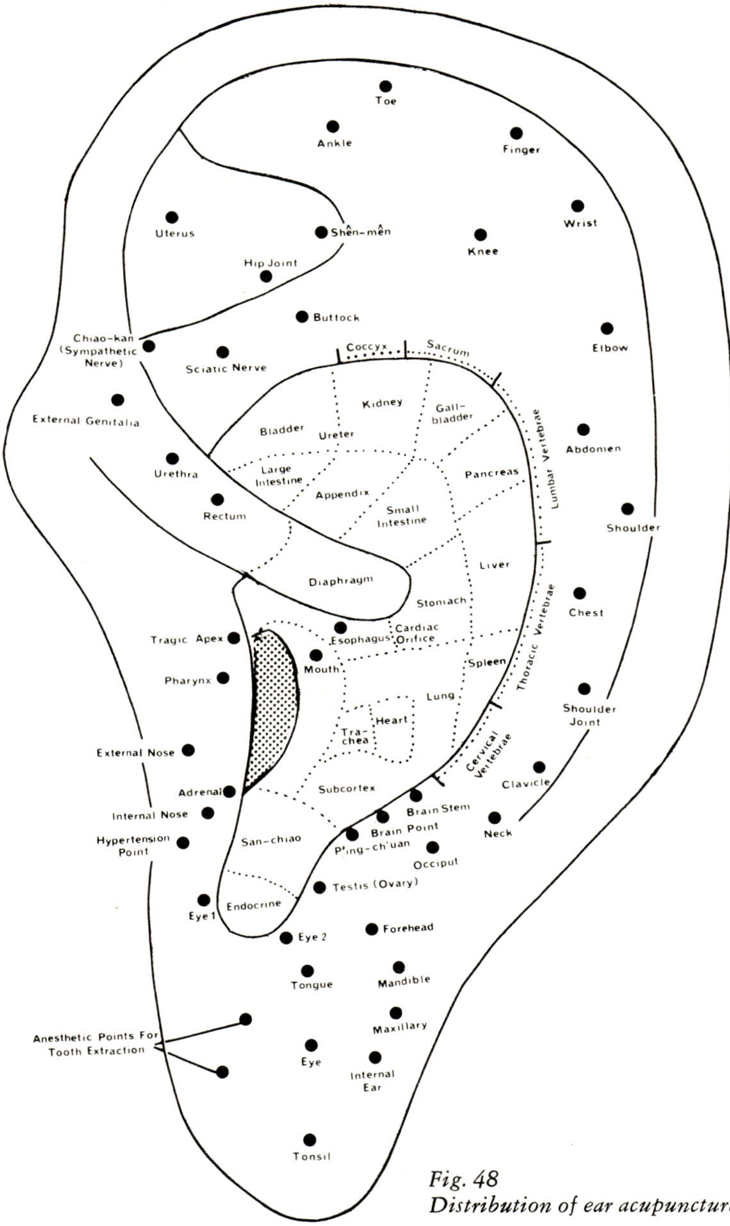

Fig. 48
Distribution of ear acupuncture points

hormonal system. For diseases of the internal organs, the specific points in both ears are used.

Technique. After the specific site of the auricle has been selected, the exact location for acupuncture is detected by:

1. Gently tapping the specific ear site with a needle to locate the most sensitive spot and thereby the acupuncture point.
2. Observing for physical changes such as discoloration (red or dark spots). In general, pain will be elicited from these discolored spots when pressure is applied to them.

Following identification of the point, a needle a half-inch long is inserted through the skin and into the cartilage but not through it. The patient should be warned of pain accompanying the needle insertion. The needle is then intermittently twirled for 15 to 30 minutes.

Table 6

LOCATION OF ACUPUNCTURE POINTS OF THE EAR
(see Fig. 48)

EAR LOCATION	NAME OF POINT
Lobule	Eye-1, Eye-2, Eye Anesthetic points for tooth extraction Internal ear Tonsil Tongue Mandible Maxillary
Antitragus	Brain Brain stem P'ing-ch'uan Subcortex Occiput Forehead Testis (ovary)
Antihelix, superior crus antihelicis, and inferior crus antihelicis	Toe Ankle Knee Sciatic nerve Buttocks Abdomen Chest Neck Coccyx Cervical, thoracic, and lumbosacral vertebrae Chiao-kan (Sympathetic nerve)
Triangular fossa	Shên-mên Uterus Hip joint
Scaphoid fossa	Finger Wrist Elbow Shoulder Shoulder joint Clavicle

Table 6 (Cont.)

EAR LOCATION	NAME OF POINT
Tragus	External nose Pharynx Internal nose Tragic apex Adrenal gland
Incisura intertragica	Endocrine system Scrotum
Inferior concha	Thorax Heart Lung Cardiac orifice Esophagus Trachea San-chiao Stomach
Superior concha	Urinary bladder Kidney Gallbladder Pancreas Liver Spleen Large intestines Small intestines Appendix
Crus helicis	Diaphragm
Helix	Rectum Urethra External genitalia Ear apex
Back of ear	Back (upper, middle, and lower) Groove for lowering blood pressure

LESS COMMONLY USED ACUPUNCTURE POINTS

3 LESS COMMONLY USED ACUPUNCTURE POINTS

More than a third of the known acupuncture points of the body have been described in the preceding chapter. They are the points most commonly used in acupuncture therapy. The remaining acupuncture points of the body comprise the contents of this section of the book. Although less frequently used, these points are also employed in acupuncture treatment either by themselves or to supplement those in chapter 2. Enumerated in tabular form, they are nevertheless described in detail with reference to nomenclature, location, indications for usage, and technique of acupuncture. Whole body charts are included to illustrate their anatomical and meridian locations.

Where indicated, appropriate acupuncture points from the preceding chapter are also listed in these tables for the purpose of maintaining meridian continuity. These points are identified by multiple asterisks (***).

Table 7

THE LUNG MERIDIAN OF HAND—TAIYIN (L)

General indications: Chest congestion, cough, dyspnea, asthma, sore throat, coryza, chills, shoulder and back pain, and pain along the course of this meridian

MERIDIAN NUMBER	NAME OF POINT	LOCATION	SPECIFIC INDICATIONS	TECHNIQUE
L 1	Chung-fu 中府	Lateral aspect of chest between the 1st and 2d ribs, 6 in. lateral to the anterior midline	Cough, dyspnea, chest pain, shoulder and back pain	Diagonally 0.5 in. towards lateral aspect of the chest
L 2	Yun-mên 云门	Below the acromial extremity of the clavicle in the depression lateral to the triangle of m. pectoralis	As above, and asthma	Diagonally 0.5 to 1.0 in. deep. Moxa heating for 5 to 15 min.
L 3	T'ien-fu 天府	Medial aspect of the upper arm, 3 in. below the anterior axillary fold on the radial side of m. biceps brachii	Epistaxis, pain in the medial aspect of the upper arm	Perpendicularly 0.5 to 1.0 in. deep. Moxa heating for 5 min.
L 4	Hsia-pai 侠白	1.0 in. below T'ien-fu	Dyspnea and pain of the upper arm	Perpendicularly 0.5 to 1.0 in. deep
L 5	Ch'ih-che 尸泽	* * *		
L 6	Kung-tsui 孔最	* * *		

L 7	Lieh-ch'üeh 列缺	* * *		
L 8	Chin-chu 经渠	1.0 in. above the most distal crease on the ventral surface of the wrist at the medial aspect of the styloid process of the radius	Pain of the hand and wrist	Perpendicularly 0.3 to 0.5 in. deep
L 9	T'ai-yüan 太渊	* * *		
L10	Yu-chi 鱼际	On the palmer surface at the center of the 1st metacarpal bone	Fever	Perpendicularly 0.3 to 0.7 in. deep. Moxa heating for 1 to 3 min.
L 11	Shao-shang 少商	* * *		

Table 8

THE LARGE INTESTINE MERIDIAN OF HAND—YANGMING (LI)

General indications: Abdominal pain, borborygmus, constipation, diarrhea, sore throat, toothache, nasal discharge, epistaxis, and pain along the course of this meridian

MERIDIAN NUMBER	NAME OF POINT	LOCATION	SPECIFIC INDICATIONS	TECHNIQUE
LI 1	Shang-yang 商阳	On the radial side of the index finger, 0.1 in. proximal to the corner of the fingernail	Fever, coma, and apoplexy	Prick till blood is drawn
LI 2	Erh-chien 二间	Immediately distal to the 2d metacarpo-phalangeal joint on the radial side. Clench fist to locate the point	Facial paralysis and fever	Perpendicularly 0.2 to 0.3 in. deep. Moxa heating for 5 min.
LI 3	San-chien 三间	On the radial side of the index finger, immediately proximal to the head of the 2d metacarpal bone	Ophthalmalgia, trigeminal neuralgia, redness and swelling of fingers and back of hand	Perpendicularly 0.3 in. deep. Moxa heating for 5 to 10 min.
LI 4	Ho-ku 合谷	* * *		
LI 5	Yang-ch'i 阳溪	* * *		

LI 6	Pian-li 偏历	3.0 in. above Yang-ch'i	Facial paralysis, tonsillitis, and edema	Perpendicularly 0.3 to 1.0 in. deep. Moxa heating for 5 to 15 min.
LI 7	Wên-liu 温溜	5.0 in. above Yang-ch'i	Stomatitis, parotitis, and glossitis	Perpendicularly 0.5 to 1.0 in. deep. Moxa heating for 5 to 15 min.
LI 8	Hsia-lien 下廉	4.0 in. below Ch'ü-ch'ih	Mastitis and pain of the elbow and arm	As above
LI 9	Shang-lien 上廉	3.0 in. below Ch'ü-ch'ih	Shoulder and back pain, and paresthesia of the upper extremities	As above
LI 10	Shou-san-li 手三里	2.0 in. below Ch'u-ch'ih	Pain of shoulder and arm, tremor, and hemiplegia	Perpendicularly 1.0 to 2.0 in. deep. Moxa heating for 5 to 15 min.
LI 11	Ch'u-ch'ih 曲池	* * *		
LI 12	Chao-liao 肘髎	* * *		
LI 13	Shou-wu-li 手五里	3.0 in. above Ch'u-ch'ih	Pneumonia, peritonitis, and pain of arm and elbow	As above

THE LARGE INTESTINE MERIDIAN OF HAND—YANGMING (Cont.)

MERIDIAN NUMBER	NAME OF POINT	LOCATION	SPECIFIC INDICATIONS	TECHNIQUE
LI 14	Pi-nao 臂臑	* * *		
LI 15	Chien-yü 肩髃	* * *		
LI 16	Chü-ku 巨骨	* * *		
LI 17	T'ien-ting 天鼎	1.0 in. below Fuh-t'u	Tonsillitis	Perpendicularly 0.5 to 1.0 in. deep. Moxa heating for 5 to 10 min.
LI 18	Fuh-t'u 扶突	* * *		
LI 19	Ho-liao 禾髎	0.5 in. lateral to Jen-chung	Facial paralysis and nasal obstruction	Diagonally 0.3 to 0.5 in. deep
LI 20	Yin-hsiang 迎香	* * *		

Table 9

THE STOMACH MERIDIAN OF FOOT—YANGMING (S)

General indications: Abdominal distention, borborygmus, gastralgia, edema, vomiting, facial paralysis, sore throat, epistaxis, chest and knee pain, fever, and mania

MERIDIAN NUMBER	NAME OF POINT	LOCATION	SPECIFIC INDICATIONS	TECHNIQUE
S 1	Ch'êng-ch'i 承泣	* * *		
S 2	Szŭ-pê 四白	* * *		
S 3	Chü-liao 巨髎	Directly below Szŭ-pê, level with the lower end of the ala nasi	Toothache, pain, and swelling of the lips and cheek	Diagonally 0.3 to 0.5 in. deep. Moxa heating for 5 min.
S 4	Ti-ts'ang 地仓	* * *		
S 5	Ta-ying 大迎	0.5 in. anterior to Chia-ch'ê	Toothache and parotitis	Perpendicularly 0.5 to 0.8 in. deep. Moxa heating for 5 to 10 min.
S 6	Chia-ch'ê 頰車	* * *		

THE STOMACH MERIDIAN OF FOOT—YANGMING (Cont.)

MERIDIAN NUMBER	NAME OF POINT	LOCATION	SPECIFIC INDICATIONS	TECHNIQUE
S 7	Hsia-kuan 下关	* * *		
S 8	Tou-wei 头維	Corner of the forehead, 0.5 in. above the hairline	Migraine, ophthalmalgia, and excessive lacrimation	Diagonally 0.3 to 0.5 in. deep
S 9	Jen-ying 人迎	1.5 in. directly lateral to the laryngeal prominence	Hypertension, asthma, and aphasia	Perpendicularly 0.5 to 1.0 in. deep
S 10	Shui-tu 水突	Anterior border of the m. sternocleidomastoideus, midway between Jen-ying and Ch'i-shu	Sore throat and asthma	Diagonally 0.5 to 1.0 in. deep. Moxa heating for 5 to 10 min.
S 11	Ch'i-shu 气舍	Directly below Jen-ying on the superior border of the clavicle	Dyspnea and torticollis	Perpendicularly 0.3 to 0.5 in. deep. Moxa heating for 5 to 15 min.
S 12	Ch'üeh-pên 缺盆	Middle of the supraclavicular fossa along the mammillary line	Asthma, pleuritis, and intercostal neuralgia	Perpendicularly 0.3 to 0.5 in. deep. Moxa heating for 5 to 10 min.
S 13	Ch'i-fu	4.0 in. lateral to Hsüan-chi	Asthma, bronchitis, dyspnea and hiccough	Diagonally 0.5 to 0.8 in. deep. Moxa

S 14	Ku-fang 庫房	1st intercostal space, 4.0 in. lateral to the anterior midline	Bronchitis	Diagonally 0.5 to 0.8 in. deep. Moxa heating for 5 to 15 min.
S 15	Wu-yi 屋翳	2d intercostal space, 4.0 in. lateral to the anterior midline	Bronchitis and asthma	As above
S 16	Ying-chuang 膺窗	3d intercostal space, 4.0 in. lateral to the anterior midline	Cough, asthma, diarrhea, mastitis, and pain in the hypochondriac region	As above
S 17	Ru-chung 乳中	4th intercostal space at the center of the nipple	Serves as a point of reference for locating points of the chest and abdomen	Not for acupuncture or moxa heating
S 18	Ru-kêng 乳根	* * *		
S 19	Pu-yung 不容	6.0 in. above the umbilicus, 2.0 in. lateral to the midline	Stomach distention and intercostal neuralgia	Perpendicularly 0.5 in. deep. Moxa heating for 5 to 20 min.
S 20	Ch'êng-man 承滿	5.0 in. above the umbilicus, 2.0 in. lateral to the midline	Gastritis and pain and spasm of the m. rectus abdominis	Perpendicularly 0.5 to 0.8 in. deep. Moxa heating for 5 to 20 min.
S 21	Lian-mên 梁门	4.0 in. above the umbilicus, 2.0 in. lateral to the midline	Gastric or duodenal ulcer and gastralgia	As above

THE STOMACH MERIDIAN OF FOOT—YANGMING (Cont.)

MERIDIAN NUMBER	NAME OF POINT	LOCATION	SPECIFIC INDICATIONS	TECHNIQUE
S 22	Kuan-mên 关门	3.0 in. above the umbilicus, 2.0 in. lateral to the midline	Anorexia, diarrhea, and edema	As above
S 23	Tai-yi 太乙	2.0 in. above the umbilicus, 2.0 in. lateral to the midline	Hernia, enuresis, and mental disorder	As above
S 24	Hua-jou-mên 滑肉门	1.0 in. above the umbilicus, 2.0 in. lateral to the midline	Nausea and mental disorder	As above
S 25	T'ien-shu 天枢	* * *		
S 26	Wai-ling 外陵	1.0 in. below the umbilicus, 2.0 in. lateral to the midline	Abdominal pain and menorrhagia	As above
S 27	Ta-chü 大巨	2.0 in. below the umbilicus, 2.0 in. lateral to the midline	Cystitis and dysentery	As above
S 28	Shui-tao 水道	3.0 in. below the umbilicus, 2.0 in. lateral to the midline	Nephritis, cystitis, orchitis, and urinary retention	As above
S 29	Kuei-lai 归来	4.0 in. below T'ien-shu, 2.0 in. lateral to the midline	Amenorrhea, menorrhagia, uterine prolapse, epididymitis, hernia, and chronic	Perpendicularly 0.5 to 1.0 in. deep. Moxa heating for 10 to 20 min.

S 30	Ch'i-ch'ung 气冲	* * *		
S 31	Pi-kuan 髀关	Directly below the anterior superior iliac spine, level with the lower border of the symphysis pubis	Paralysis of the lower extremities and rheumatism	Perpendicularly 1.0 to 1.5 in. deep. Moxa heating for 5 to 10 min.
S 32	Fu-t'u 伏兔	* * *		
S 33	Yin-shih 阴市	3.0 in. above the superior and lateral border of the patella	Pain of the knee joint and paralysis of the lower limbs	As above
S 34	Liang-ch'iu 梁丘	* * *		
S 35	Tu-pi 犊鼻	It is the lateral point of Nei-wai-ch'i-yen		
S 36	Tsu-san-li 足三里	* * *		
S 37	Shang-chü-hsü 上巨虚	* * *		
S 38	Tiao-kou 条口	8.0 in. below the knee, 2.0 in. below Shang-chu-hsu	Paralysis or pain of the lower extremities and arthritis of the shoulder	Perpendicularly 1.0 to 1.5 in. deep. Moxa heating for 5 to 20 min.

THE STOMACH MERIDIAN OF FOOT—YANGMING (Cont.)

MERIDIAN NUMBER	NAME OF POINT	LOCATION	SPECIFIC INDICATIONS	TECHNIQUE
S 39	Hsia-chü-hsü 下巨虚	3.0 in. distal to Shang-chü-hsü	Paralysis of the lower limbs and abdominal pain	Perpendicularly 1.0 in. deep. Moxa heating for 5 to 20 min.
S 40	Fêng-lung 丰隆	* * *		
S 41	Chiai-ch'i 解溪	* * *		
S 42	Ch'ung-yang 冲阳	1.5 in. distal to Chiai-ch'i	Pain in dorsum of foot, paralysis of the lower extremities, toothache, gingivitis, and epilepsy	Perpendicularly 0.3 to 0.5 in. deep. Moxa heating for 5 to 10 min.
S 43	Hsien-ku 陷谷	* * *		
S 44	Nei-ting 内庭	* * *		
S 45	Li-tui 厉兑	Lateral side of the tip of the 2d toe, 0.1 in. posterior to the corner of the toenail.	Fever and epilepsy	Diagonally 0.1 in. deep. Moxa heating for 3 min.

Table 10

THE SPLEEN MERIDIAN OF FOOT—TAIYIN (SP)

General indications: Pain of the tongue, gastralgia, abdominal distention, emesis, jaundice, general weakness, and pain and swelling along the course of this meridian

MERIDIAN NUMBER	NAME OF POINT	LOCATION	SPECIFIC INDICATIONS	TECHNIQUE
Sp 1	Yin-pê 隐白	* * *		
Sp 2	Ta-tu 大都	At the medial aspect of the 1st toe, immediately distal to the metatarso-phalangeal joint	Fever and hypohydrosis	Perpendicularly 0.3 to 0.5 in. deep. Moxa heating for 15 to 20 min.
Sp 3	Tai-pê 太白	At the medial aspect of the foot, immediately proximal to the 1st metatarso-phalangeal joint	Dysentery and constipation	Perpendicularly 0.3 to 0.5 in. deep. Moxa heating for 5 to 10 min.
Sp 4	Kung-sun 公孙	* * *		
Sp 5	Shang-ch'iu 商丘	* * *		
Sp 6	San-yin-chiao 三阴交	* * *		

THE SPLEEN MERIDIAN OF FOOT—TAIYIN (Cont.)

MERIDIAN NUMBER	NAME OF POINT	LOCATION	SPECIFIC INDICATIONS	TECHNIQUE
Sp 7	Lou-ku 漏谷	3.0 in. above San-yin-chiao at the posterior border of the tibia	Borborygmus and numbness of the leg and knee	Perpendicularly 1.0 to 1.5 in. deep. Moxa heating for 5 to 10 min.
Sp 8	Ti-chi 地机	3.0 in. below Yin-lin-ch'üan at the posterior border of the tibia	Lumbago and menorrhagia	Perpendicularly 1.0 to 2.0 in. deep. Moxa heating for 5 to 15 min.
Sp 9	Yin-lin-ch'üan 阴陵泉	* * *		
Sp 10	Hsüeh-hai 血海	* * *		
Sp 11	Chi-mên 箕门	6.0 in. above Hsüeh-hai, medial to the m. sartorius	Dysuria, enuresis, inflammation of the inguinal lymph nodes	Perpendicularly 1.0 to 1.5 in. deep. Moxa heating for 3 to 10 min.
Sp 12	Ch'ung-mên 冲门	3.5 in. lateral to the midpoint of the superior border of the symphysis pubis	Orchitis, endometritis, and hernia	Perpendicularly 0.7 to 1.0 in. deep. Moxa heating for 10 to 20 min.

Sp 13	Fu-shu 府舍	0.7 in. above Ch'ung-mên, 4.0 in. lateral to the midline	Appendicitis and constipation	As above
Sp 14	Fu-chieh 腹结	3.0 in. above Fu-shu, 4.0 in. lateral to the midline	Periumbilical pain, hernia, and diarrhea	Perpendicularly 0.5 to 1.0 in. deep. Moxa heating for 10 to 20 min.
Sp 15	Ta-heng 大横	4.0 in. lateral to the umbilicus	Dyspepsia, constipation, paralytic ileus, and diarrhea	As above
Sp 16	Fu-ai 腹哀	3.0 in. above Ta-heng, 4.0 in. lateral to the midline	Dyspepsia, constipation, and diarrhea	As above
Sp 17	Shih-tou 食竇	5th intercostal space, 6.0 in. lateral to the midline	Pain of the chest and hypochondriac regions	Diagonally 0.5 in. deep. Moxa heating for 5 to 15 min.
Sp 18	T'ien-ch'i 天溪	4th intercostal space, 6.0 in. lateral to the midline	Chest pain, cough, and mastitis	As above
Sp 19	Hsiung-hsiang 胸乡	3d intercostal space, 6.0 in. lateral to the midline	Pain of the chest and hypochondriac regions	As above
Sp 20	Chou-jung 周荣	2d intercostal space, 6.0 in. lateral to the midline	Cough, pain of the chest and hypochondriac regions	As above
Sp 21	Ta-pao 大包	6th intercostal space, at the midaxillary line	Chest pain, dyspnea, generalized bodyaches	Diagonally 0.5 in. deep. Moxa heating for 10 to 20 min.

Table 11

THE HEART MERIDIAN OF HAND—SHAOYIN (H)

General indications: Dryness of the throat, pain in the cardiac and hypochondriac regions, thirst, jaundice, and pain along the course of this meridian

MERIDIAN NUMBER	NAME OF POINT	LOCATION	SPECIFIC INDICATIONS	TECHNIQUE
H 1	Chi-ch'üan 极泉	* * *		
H 2	Ching-ling 青灵	3.0 in. above the elbow, medial to the m. biceps brachii	Pain of the shoulder and arm	Perpendicularly 0.5 to 1.0 in. deep. Moxa heating for 5 to 10 min.
H 3	Shao-hai 少海	* * *		
H 4	Ling-tao 灵道	1.5 in. above Shên-mên	Angina pectoris, ulnar neuralgia, and hysteria	Perpendicularly 0.3 to 0.5 in. deep. Moxa heating for 10 to 20 min.
H 5	Tung-li 通里	1.0 in. above Shên-mên	Acute hoarseness of voice, asphasia, insomnia, palpitation, and arm and wrist pain	As above

H 6	Yin-hsi 阴郄	0.5 in. above Shên-mên	Neurasthenia, angina pectoris, palpitation, and night sweats	As above
H 7	Shên-mên 神门	* * *		
H 8	Shao-fu 少府	On the palmar surface, between the 4th and 5th metacarpal bones and also between the tips of the 4th and 5th fingers when making a fist	Palpitation, chest pain, pruritus vulvae, dysuria, and enuresis	Perpendicularly 0.3 to 0.5 in. deep
H 9	Shao-ch'ung 少冲	On the radial side of the tip of the 5th finger, 0.1 in. proximal to the corner of the fingernail	Palpitation, chest pain, apoplexy, and coma	Perpendicularly 0.1 in. deep

Table 12

THE SMALL INTESTINE MERIDIAN OF HAND—TAIYANG (SI)

General indications: Pain in the lower abdomen, deafness, jaundice, swelling of the cheek, sore throat, and pain along the course of the meridian

MERIDIAN NUMBER	NAME OF POINT	LOCATION	SPECIFIC INDICATIONS	TECHNIQUE
SI 1	Shao-che 少泽	* * *		
SI 2	Chien-ku 前谷	0.5 in. distal to Hou-ch'i	Fever, eye diseases, tinnitus, and numbness of the fingers	Perpendicularly 0.2 to 0.3 in. deep. Moxa heating for 5 to 10 min.
SI 3	Hou-ch'i 后溪	* * *		
SI 4	Wan-ku 腕骨	At the ulnar border of the palm between the base of the 5th metacarpal bone and the trigonal bone	Arthritis of the elbow, wrist, and finger joints, headache, tinnitus, emesis, and cholecystitis	Perpendicularly 0.3 to 0.5 in. deep. Moxa heating for 5 to 20 min.
SI 5	Yang-ku 阳谷	At the ulnar side of the wrist between the styloid process of the ulna and the pisiform bone	Mental disorder, tinnitus, and arm and wrist pain	As above

SI 6	Yang-lao 养老	With the forearm flexed and the palm placed on the chest, the point is at the bony cleft on the radial aspect of the styloid process of the ulna	Visual impairment, paralysis of the upper extremities, and pain of the wrist	Diagonally towards Nei-kuan, and 1.0 to 1.5 in. deep. Moxa heating for 5 to 10 min.
SI 7	Chih-cheng 支正	5.0 in. above Yang-ku	Torticollis and mental disorder	Perpendicularly 0.5 to 0.8 in. deep. Moxa heating for 5 to 15 min.
SI 8	Hsiao-hai 小海	With the forearm flexed, it is between the olecranon of the ulna and the tip of the medial epicondyle of the humerus	Pain of the small finger, elbow, shoulder, and back	Perpendicularly 0.3 to 0.5 in. deep. Moxa heating for 5 to 15 min.
SI 9	Chien-chên 肩貞	* * *		
SI 10	Nao-yü 臑俞	* * *		
SI 11	T'ien-tsung 天宗	* * *		
SI 12	Ping-fêng 秉风	In the center of the suprascapular fossa	Pain and numbness of the shoulder joint and upper extremities	Diagonally 0.5 to 1.0 in. deep. Moxa heating for 5 to 15 min.
SI 13	Ch'u-yüan 曲垣	* * *		

THE SMALL INTESTINE MERIDIAN OF HAND—TAIYANG (Cont.)

NUMBER MERIDIAN	NAME OF POINT	LOCATION	SPECIFIC INDICATIONS	TECHNIQUE
SI 14	Chien-wai-yü 肩外俞	3.0 in. lateral to the lower border of the spinous process of the 1st thoracic vertebra	Pain of the neck and scapular joint and torticollis	As above
SI 15	Chien-chung-yü 肩中俞	2.0 in. lateral to the lower border of the spinous process of the 7th cervical vertebra	Pain and stiffness of the neck, shoulder and back, bronchitis, and asthma	As above
SI 16	T'ien-chuang 天窗	At the posterior border of the m. sternocleidomastoideus, 0.5 in. posterior to Fuh-t'u	Tinnitus and torticollis	Perpendicularly 0.5 to 1.0 in. deep. Moxa heating for 5 to 10 min.
SI 17	T'ien-yung 天容	* * *		
SI 18	Chuan-liao 顴髎	* * *		
SI 19	T'ing-kung 听宫	* * *		

Table 13

THE BLADDER MERIDIAN OF FOOT—TAIYANG (BL)

General indications: Urinary retention, enuresis, mania, headache, eye diseases, pain of the upper and lower back and the lower extremities

MERIDIAN NUMBER	NAME OF POINT	LOCATION	SPECIFIC INDICATIONS	TECHNIQUE
Bl 1	Ching-ming 睛明	* * *		
Bl 2	Tsuan-tsu 攢竹	* * *		
Bl 3	Mei-ch'ung 眉冲	Directly above Tsuan-tsu, 0.5 in. above the hairline	Excessive lacrimation and leucoma	Diagonally 0.3 to 0.5 in. deep
Bl 4	Ch'u-cha 曲差	0.5 in. lateral to Mei-ch'ung	Nasal obstruction and epistaxis	Diagonally 0.3 to 0.5 in. deep. Moxa heating for 5 to 15 min.
Bl 5	Wu-chu 五处	0.5 in. above Ch'u-cha	Epilepsy	As above
Bl 6	Ch'êng-kuang 承光	1.5 in. posterior to Wu-chu	Dizziness, leucoma, and coryza	Diagonally 0.3 to 0.5 in. deep
Bl 7	T'ung-t'ien 通天	* * *		

THE BLADDER MERIDIAN OF FOOT—TAIYANG (Cont.)

MERIDIAN NUMBER	NAME OF POINT	LOCATION	SPECIFIC INDICATIONS	TECHNIQUE
Bl 8	Lo-ch'üeh 络郄	1.5 in. posterior to T'ung-t'ien	Rhinitis, epistaxis, headache (vertex), and bronchitis	Diagonally 0.3 to 0.5 in. deep. Moxa heating for 5 to 15 min.
Bl 9	Yü-chen 玉枕	Lateral side of the superior border of the external occipital protuberance, 1.3 in. lateral to the midline	Dizziness, myopia, and headache (vertex)	As above
Bl 10	T'ien-chu 天柱	* * *		
Bl 11	Ta-shu 大杼	1.5in. lateral to the midline, at a level between the 1st and 2d thoracic vertebrae	Cough, fever, and pain of the shoulder joint	Diagonally 0.3 to 0.5 in. deep
Bl 12	Fêng-mên 风门	* * *		
Bl 13	Fei-yü 肺俞	* * *		
Bl 14	Chueh-yin-yü 厥阴俞	1.5 in. lateral to the midline at a level between the 4th and 5th vertebrae	Neurasthenia, headache (vertex), hiccough, chest pain, and pericarditis	Diagonally 0.3 to 0.5 in. deep and caudad. Moxa heating for 5 to 15 min.

Bl 15	Hsin-yü 心俞	* * *		
Bl 16	Tu-yü 督俞	1.5 in. lateral to the midline at a level between the 6th and 7th thoracic vertebrae	Endocarditis, hiccough, borborygmus, and pruritus	As above
Bl 17	Ke-yü 膈俞	* * *		
Bl 18	Kan-yü 肝俞	* * *		
Bl 19	Tan-yü 胆俞	* * *		
Bl 20	P'i-yü 脾俞	* * *		
Bl 21	Wei-yü 胃俞	* * *		
Bl 22	San-jiao-yü 三焦俞	1.5 in. lateral to the midline at a level between the 1st and 2d lumbar vertebrae	Gastralgia, dyspepsia, enteritis, nephritis, neurasthenia, lumbago, and enuresis	Perpendicularly 0.5 to 1.0 in. deep. Moxa heating for 5 to 20 min.
Bl 23	Shêng-yü 腎俞	* * *		
Bl 24	Ch'i-hai-yü 气海俞	* * *		

THE BLADDER MERIDIAN OF FOOT—TAIYANG (Cont.)

MERIDIAN NUMBER	NAME OF POINT	LOCATION	SPECIFIC INDICATIONS	TECHNIQUE
Bl 25	Ta-ch'ang-yü 大肠俞	* * *		
Bl 26	Kuan-yüan-yü 关元俞	1.5 in. lateral to the midline at a level between the 5th lumbar and 1st sacral vertebrae	Lumbago, diarrhea, and urogenital diseases	Perpendicularly 1.0 to 1.5 in. deep. Moxa heating for 5 to 20 min.
Bl 27	Hsiao-ch'ang-yü 小肠俞	* * *		
Bl 28	P'ang-k'uang-yü 膀胱俞	* * *		
Bl 29	Chung-lu-yü 中膂俞	1.5 in. lateral to the midline at the level of the 3d sacral foramen	Enteritis, lumbago, and sciatica	As above
Bl 30	Pê-huan-yü 白环俞	1.5 in. lateral to the midline at the level of the 4th sacral foramen	Sciatica, hernia, leukorrhea, prostatorrhea, and endometritis	As above
Bl 31	Shang-liao 上髎	* * *		

Bl 32	Ts'ŭ-liao 次髎	* * *		
Bl 33	Chung-liao 中髎	1.0 in. lateral to the midline at the 3d sacral foramen	Menstrual irregularity, urinary problems, sciatica, and low backache	As above
Bl 34	Hsia-liao 下髎	1.0 in. lateral to the midline at the 4th sacral foramen	Same as Chung-liao	As above
Bl 35	Hui-yang 会阳	0.5 in. lateral to the midline lateral to the lower end of the coccyx	Leukorrhea, impotence, diarrhea, and hemorrhoids	Perpendicularly 1.0 to 1.5 in. deep
Bl 36	Ch'êng-fu 承扶	* * *		
Bl 37	Yin-mên 殷门	* * *		
Bl 38	Fu-hsi 浮郄	1.0 in above Wei-yang	Cystitis, constipation, dysuria, and paralysis of the lower extremities	Perpendicularly 1.0 to 1.5 in. deep. Moxa heating for 5 to 20 min.
Bl 39	Wei-yang 委阳	At the lateral point of the popliteal crease lateral to Wei-chung	Back pain, and spasm of the m. gastrocnemius	Perpendicularly 0.5 to 1.0 in. deep. Moxa heating for 3 to 5 min.
Bl 40	Wei-chung 委中	* * *		

THE BLADDER MERIDIAN OF FOOT—TAIYANG (Cont.)

MERIDIAN NUMBER	NAME OF POINT	LOCATION	SPECIFIC INDICATIONS	TECHNIQUE
Bl 41	Fu-fên 附分	3.0 in. lateral to the midline level with the spinous process of the 2d thoracic vertebra	Intercostal neuralgia and numbness of the elbow and arm	Diagonally 0.3 to 0.5 in. deep. Moxa heating for 10 to 20 min.
Bl 42	Po-hu 魄户	3.0 in. lateral to the spinous process of the 3d thoracic vertebra	Bronchitis, asthma, pleuritis, emesis, and shoulder pain	Diagonally 0.3 to 0.5 in. deep. Moxa heating for 10 to 20 min.
Bl 43	Kao-mang 膏肓	3.0 in. lateral to the spinous process of the 4th thoracic vertebra	Bronchitis, pleuritis, neurasthenia, and general weakness	As above
Bl 44	Shên-tang 神堂	3.0 in. lateral to the spinous process of the 5th thoracic vertebra	Bronchitis, asthma, cardiac diseases, and shoulder and back pain	As above
Bl 45	Yi-hsi 噫嘻	3.0 in. lateral to the spinous process of the 6th thoracic vertebra	Pericarditis, hiccough, emesis, dizziness, and asthma	As above
Bl 46	Ke-kuan 膈关	3.0 in. lateral to the spinous process of the 7th thoracic vertebra	Intercostal neuralgia, hiccough, and emesis	As above
Bl 47	Hun-mên	3.0 in. lateral to the spinous	Liver diseases, gastral-	Diagonally 0.3 to 0.5

Bl 48	Yang-kang 阳纲	3.0 in. lateral to the spinous process of the 10th thoracic vertebra	Diarrhea, borborygmus, abdominal pain, and jaundice	As above
Bl 49	Yi-she 意舍	3.0 in. lateral to the spinous process of the 11th thoracic vertebra	Dyspepsia, emesis, liver diseases, and back pain	As above
Bl 50	Wei-chang 胃仓	3.0 in. lateral to the spinous process of the 12th thoracic vertebra	Gastralgia, emesis, abdominal distention, and back pain	As above
Bl 51	Mang-mên 肓门	3.0 in. lateral to the spinous process of the 1st lumbar vertebra	Constipation, upper abdominal pain, and mastitis	Perpendicularly 0.5 to 1.0 in. deep. Moxa heating for 10 to 20 min.
Bl 52	Chih-shih 志室	* * *		
Bl 53	Pao-mang 胞肓	3.0 in. lateral to the midline, at the level of the 2d sacral foramen	Enteritis, abdominal distention, and low back pain	Perpendicularly 1.0 to 1.5 in. deep. Moxa heating for 10 to 20 min.
Bl 54	Chih-pien 秩边	* * *		
Bl 55	Ho-yang 合阳	2.0 in. directly below Wei-chung	Lumbago, leg pain, and paralysis of the lower extremities	As above
Bl 56	Ch'êng-chin 承筋	Midway between Ho-yang and Ch'eng-san	Headache, leg pain, hemorrhoids, and low back pain	As above

THE BLADDER MERIDIAN OF FOOT—TAIYANG (Cont.)

MERIDIAN NUMBER	NAME OF POINT	LOCATION	SPECIFIC INDICATIONS	TECHNIQUE
Bl 57	Ch'êng-san 承山	* * *		
Bl 58	Fei-yang 飞扬	7.0 in. above K'un-lun, posterior to the external malleolus	Ophthalmalgia, leg pain, nephritis, cystitis, and lumbago	Perpendicularly 1.0 to 1.5 in. deep. Moxa heating for 5 to 20 min.
Bl 59	Fu-yang 跗阳	3.0 in. above K'un-lun, posterior to the external malleolus	Headache and pain of the lumbosacral and ankle regions	Perpendicularly 0.5 to 1.0 in. deep. Moxa heating for 5 to 15 min.
Bl 60	K'un-lun 昆仑	* * *		
Bl 61	Pu-shên 仆参	1.5 in. inferior to the external malleolus, directly below K'un-lun	Painful heel and paralysis of the lower extremities	Perpendicularly 0.3 to 0.5 in. deep. Moxa heating for 5 to 15 min.
Bl 62	Shên-mo 申脉	Directly and immediately below the tip of the external malleolus	Headache, dizziness, epilepsy, and pain of the ankle	Perpendicularly 0.3 to 0.5 in. deep. Moxa heating for 3 to 5 min.

Bl 63	Chin-mên 金门	Posterior to the tuberosity of the 5th metatarsal bone	Lumbago, convulsions, and pain of the leg and ankle	Perpendicularly 0.3 to 0.5 in. deep. Moxa heating for 5 to 15 min.
Bl 64	Ching-ku 京骨	Below the tuberosity of the 5th metatarsal bone	Headache, epilepsy, lumbago, and leg pain	As above
Bl 65	Shu-ku 束骨	* * *		
Bl 66	Tung-ku 通谷	Immediately distal and lateral to the 5th metatarso-phalangeal joint	Headache, dizziness, epistaxis, and dyspepsia	Perpendicularly 0.2 to 0.3 in. deep. Moxa heating for 5 to 20 min.
Bl 67	Chih-yin 至阴	* * *		

Table 14

THE KIDNEY MERIDIAN OF FOOT—SHAOYIN (K)

General indications: Dyspnea, hemoptysis, sore throat, lumbago, edema, constipation, diarrhea, paralysis of the lower extremities, and pain along the path of this meridian

MERIDIAN NUMBER	NAME OF POINT	LOCATION	SPECIFIC INDICATIONS	TECHNIQUE
K 1	Yung-ch'üan 涌泉	* * *		
K 2	Jan-ku 然谷	At the instep of the foot immediately distal to the navicular bone	Cystitis, diabetes, and menstrual irregularity	Perpendicularly 0.5 to 1.0 in. deep. Moxa heating for 5 to 10 min.
K 3	T'ai-ch'i 太溪	* * *		
K 4	Ta-chung 大鈡	0.5 in. slightly posterior and distal to T'ai-ch'i	Neurasthenia, painful heel, hysteria, dysuria, and asthma	Perpendicularly 0.3 to 0.5 in. deep. Moxa heating for 5 to 20 min.
K 5	Shui-ch'üan 水泉	1.0 in. directly distal to T'ai-ch'i	Menstrual irregularity, uterine prolapse, dysuria, and myopia	As above
K 6	Chao-hai 照海	1.0 in. directly below the tip of the medial malleolus	Menstrual irregularity, uterine prolapse, epilepsy, and tonsillitis	As above

K 7	Fu-liu 复溜	* * *		
K 8	Chiao-hsin 交信	2.0 in. above T'ai-ch'i and 0.5 in. anterior to Fu-liu and posterior to the tibia	Menstrual irregularity, uterine bleeding, pain of testis	Perpendicularly 0.5 to 1.0 in deep. Moxa heating for 5 to 20 min.
K 9	Chu-pin 筑宾	5.0 in. above T'ai-ch'i and 1.0 in. posterior to the tibia	Gastrocnemius spasm, epilepsy, mental disorder, and kidney and bladder infections	Perpendicularly 1.0 to 1.5 in. deep. Moxa heating for 5 to 15 min.
K 10	Yin-ku 阴谷	At the medial end of the popliteal transverse crease between the tendons of m. semitendinosus and m. semimembranosus	Knee pain, abdominal pain, and disorders of the genital system	Perpendicularly 0.8 to 1.0 in. deep. Moxa heating for 5 to 10 min.
K 11	Hêng-ku 横骨	On the superior border of the pubic symphysis, 0.5 in. lateral to the midline	Enuresis, dysuria, hernia, prostatorrhea, and impotence	Perpendicularly 0.5 to 1.0 in. deep. Moxa heating for 10 to 20 min.
K 12	Ta-hên 大赫	1.0 in. above Hêng-ku, 0.5 in. lateral to the midline	Prostatorrhea, pain in the external genitalia, and excessive leukorrhea	As above
K 13	Ch'i-hsüeh 气穴	2.0 in. above Hêng-ku, 0.5 in. lateral to the midline	Menstrual irregularity and diarrhea	As above
K 14	Szŭ-man 四满	3.0 in. above Hêng-ku, 0.5 in. lateral to the midline	Menstrual irregularity, diarrhea, and abdominal pain	As above

THE KIDNEY MERIDIAN OF FOOT—SHAOYIN (Cont.)

MERIDIAN NUMBER	NAME OF POINT	LOCATION	SPECIFIC INDICATIONS	TECHNIQUE
K 15	Chung-zhu 中注	1.0 in. below the umbilicus, 0.5 in. lateral to the midline	Menstrual irregularity and lower abdominal pain	As above
K 16	Huang-yü 肓俞	0.5 in. lateral to the imbilicus	Jaundice, gastralgia, hernia, and menorrhagia	As above
K 17	Shang-ch'ü 商曲	2.0 in. above the umbilicus, 0.5 in. lateral to the midline	Gastralgia, hernia, abdominal pain, and anorexia	As above
K 18	Shih-kuan 石关	3.0 in. above the umbilicus, 0.5 in. lateral to the midline	Gastralgia, hiccough, and constipation	As above
K 19	Yin-tu 阴都	4.0 in. above the umbilicus, 0.5 in. lateral to the midline	Borborygmus, abdominal distention and pain	Perpendicularly 0.5 to 1.0 in. deep. Moxa heating for 10 to 20 min.
K 20	Tun-ku 通谷	5.0 in. above the umbilicus, 0.5 in. lateral to the midline	Emesis, diarrhea, abdominal distention and pain	As above
K 21	Yu-mên 幽门	6.0 in. above the umbilicus, 0.5 in. lateral to the midline	Chest pain, emesis, diarrhea, and belching	As above
K 22	Pu-lang	At the 5th intercostal space, 2.0	Intercostal neuralgia,	Diagonally 0.5 to 0.8

K 23	Shên-fêng 神封	At the 4th intercostal space, 2.0 in. lateral to the midline	Intercostal neuralgia, pleuritis, mastitis, and bronchitis	As above
K 24	Ling-hsü 灵墟	At the 3d intercostal space, 2.0 in. lateral to the midline	Intercostal neuralgia, emesis, cough, and mastitis	As above
K 25	Shên-tsang 神藏	At the 2d intercostal space, 2.0 in. lateral to the midline	Intercostal neuralgia, emesis, and cough	As above
K 26	Yu-chung 彧中	At the 1st intercostal space, 2.0 in. lateral to the midline	As above	As above
K 27	Yü-fu 俞府	Between the 1st rib and the clavicle, 2.0 in. lateral to the midline	Chest pain, asthma, emesis, and bronchitis	As above

Table 15

THE CIRCULATION-SEX (PERICARDIUM) MERIDIAN OF HAND—JUEYIN (CS)

General indications: Chest congestion, palpitation, angina pectoris, irritability and restlessness, mania, spasm of the elbow and the arm, and pain along the path of this meridian

MERIDIAN NUMBER	NAME OF POINT	LOCATION	SPECIFIC INDICATIONS	TECHNIQUE
CS 1	T'ien-chi'h 天池	4th intercostal space, 1.0 in. lateral to the nipple	Chest congestion and pain in the hypochondriac region	Diagonally 0.5 to 0.8 in. deep
CS 2	T'ien-ch'üan 天泉	Between the 2 heads of m. biceps brachii, 2 in. distal to the anterior end of the axillary fold	Chest pain, cough, and pain in the hypochondriac region, the back, and the medial aspect of the arm	Perpendicularly 1.0 to 1.5 in. deep
CS 3	Ch'ü-che 曲泽	In the antecubital fossa at the medial or ulnar side of the tendon of the biceps	Fever, palpitation, angina pectoris, and gastralgia	Perpendicularly 0.5 to 1.0 in. deep till blood is drawn. Moxa heating for 5 to 15 min.
CS 4	Hsi-mên 郄门	* * *		
CS 5	Chien-shih 间使	* * *		

CS 6	Nei-kuan 内关			
CS 7	Ta-lin 大陵	* * *		
CS 8	Lao-kung 劳宫	* * *		
CS 9	Chung-ch'ung 中冲	At the midpoint of the tip of the middle finger	Coma, apoplexy, heat stroke, and fever	Perpendicularly 0.1 in. deep till blood is drawn

Table 16

THE TRIPLE WARMER (SANJIAO) MERIDIAN OF HAND—SHAOYANG (T)

General indications: Abdominal distention, edema, enuresis, dysuria, deafness, tinnitus, sore throat, pain behind the ear, shoulder, arm, lateral aspect of the elbow, and along the course of this meridian, and swelling of cheek

MERIDIAN NUMBER	NAME OF POINT	LOCATION	SPECIFIC INDICATIONS	TECHNIQUE
T 1	Kuan-ch'ung 关 冲	0.1 in. proximal to the corner of the finger nail at the ulnar side of the 4th finger	Headache, sore throat, and fever	Diagonally 0.1 in. deep till blood is drawn
T 2	Ye-mên 液 门	Between the 4th and 5th fingers, 0.5 in. proximal to the margin of the web between the fingers	Headache, conjunctivitis, sore throat, malaria, deafness, and pain of the hand and the arm	Diagonally 0.3 to 0.5 in. deep
T 3	Chung-chu 中 渚	* * *		
T 4	Yang-ch'ih 阳 池	* * *		
T 5	Wai-kuan 外 关	* * *		
T 6	Chih-kou 支 沟	* * *		

T 7	Hui-tsung 会宗	On the radial side of the ulna 1 finger's width lateral to Chih-kou	Epilepsy, deafness, and pain of the upper extremities	Perpendicularly 0.5 to 1.0 in. deep
T 8	San-yang-lo 三阳络	* * *		
T 9	Szŭ-tu 四渎	Between the radius and the ulna, 5 in. distal to the olecranon, on the dorsum of the forearm	Toothache, deafness, and pain of the forearm	Perpendicularly 0.5 to 1.0 in. deep. Moxa heating for 5 to 10 min.
T 10	T'ien-ching 天井	* * *		
T 11	Ching-leng-yüan 清冷渊	1.0 in. above T'ien-ching with the elbow flexed	Pain in the shoulder and the arm	Perpendicularly 0.5 to 0.7 in. deep. Moxa heating for 5 to 10 min.
T 12	Hsiao-lo 消濼	Midway between Ching-leng-yüan and Nao-hui	Headache and pain in the arm	As above
T 13	Nao-hui 臑会	3.0 in. below Chien-liao at the posterior border of m. deltoideus	Eye diseases and pain of the shoulder, the arm, and the scapular joint	As above
T 14	Chien-liao 肩髎	* * *		
T 15	T'ien-liao 天髎	Midway between the tip of the acromion and Ta-ch'ui	Pain in the neck and the shoulder and paralysis of the arm	As above

THE TRIPLE WARMER MERIDIAN OF HAND—SHAOYANG (Cont.)

MERIDIAN NUMBER	NAME OF POINT	LOCATION	SPECIFIC INDICATIONS	TECHNIQUE
T 16	T'ien-yu 天牖	* * *		
T 17	I-fêng 翳风	* * *		
T 18	Chih-mo 瘈脉	At the center of the mastoid process	Deafness, facial paralysis, and tinnitus	Diagonally 0.2 to 0.3 in. deep. Moxa heating for 5 to 10 min.
T 19	Lu-hsi 颅息	1.0 in. above Chih-mo	Tinnitus, emesis, and otitis media	As above
T 20	Chiao-sun 角孙	Immediately above the superior tip of the ear	Ear inflammation, toothache, and cloudiness of the cornea	As above
T 21	Êrh-mên 耳门	* * *		
T 22	Ho-liao 和髎	On the hairline, anterior and superior to Êrh-mên	Headache, tinnitus, facial paralysis, and lockjaw	As above
T 23	Szŭ-tsu-k'ung	* * *		

Table 17

THE GALLBLADDER MERIDIAN OF FOOT—SHAOYANG (GB)

Genral indications: Dizziness, headache, bitter taste in the mouth, malaria, deafness, tinnitus, and pain in the submaxillary and outer canthus areas and along this meridian

MERIDIAN NUMBER	NAME OF POINT	LOCATION	SPECIFIC INDICATIONS	TECHNIQUE
GB 1	T'ung-tsŭ-liao 瞳子髎	* * *		
GB 2	T'ing-hui 听会	* * *		
GB 3	Shang-kuan 上关	At the upper border of the zygomatic arch directly above Hsia-kuan	Tinnitus, deafness, facial paralysis, and toothache	Perpendicularly 0.5 to 1.0 in. deep. Moxa heating for 3 to 5 min.
GB 4	Han-yên 頷厌	1.0 in. below Tou-wei at the hairline of the temporal region	Migraine, dizziness, tinnitus, rhinitis, and facial paralysis	Diagonally 0.3 to 0.5 in. deep. Moxa heating for 5 to 10 min.
GB 5	Hsuan-lu 悬顱	At the junction of the anterior and middle third of a line connecting Han-yên and Ch'ü-pin	Migraine, neurasthenia, and toothache	Diagonally 0.2 to 0.3 in. deep. Moxa heating for 5 to 10 min.

THE GALLBLADDER MERIDIAN OF FOOT—SHAOYANG (Cont.)

MERIDIAN NUMBER	NAME OF POINT	LOCATION	SPECIFIC INDICATIONS	TECHNIQUE
GB 6	Hsuan-li 悬厘	At the junction of the inferior and middle third of a line connecting Han-yên and Ch'ü-pin	Migraine, neurasthenia, facial edema, and toothache	As above
GB 7	Ch'ü-pin 曲鬓	At the hairline directly above the most anterior point of the ear	Pain of the cheek and submaxillary area, torticollis, and headache	As above
GB 8	Shuai-ku 率谷	* * *		
GB 9	T'ien-ch'ung 天冲	0.5 in. posterior to Shuai-ku	Headache, gingivitis, and epilepsy	Diagonally 0.5 to 0.8 in. deep. Moxa heating for 5 to 15 min.
GB 10	Fu-pê 浮白	1.0 in. below T'ien-ch'ung at the posterior border of the ear	Tinnitus, deafness, toothache, and tonsillitis	As above
GB 11	Tou-chiao-yin 头窍阴	Midpoint of the line connecting Fu-pê and Wan-ku	Opthalmalgia and headache (vertex)	Diagonally 0.5 to 0.8 in. deep. Moxa heating for 5 to 15 min.
GB 12	Wan-ku 完骨	In the depression immediately posterior and inferior to the	Tinnitus, toothache, facial paralysis, and	As above

GB 13	Pên-shên 本神	0.5 in. above the hairline, directly above the outer canthus	Torticollis and epilepsy	As above
GB 14	Yang-pê 阳白	* * *		
GB 15	Lin-ch'i 临泣	0.5 in. above the hairline, directly above the pupil	Nasal obstruction, eye diseases, apoplexy, and epilepsy	As above
GB 16	Mu-chuang 目窗	1.0 in. above Lin-ch'i	Eye diseases and facial edema	As above
GB 17	Cheng-ying 正营	1.0 in. posterior to Mu-chuang	Headache and toothache	As above
GB 18	Ch'êng-ling 承灵	1.5 in. posterior to Cheng-ying	Epistaxis, nasal obstruction, and headache	As above
GB 19	Nao-kung 脑空	1.5 in. above Fêng-ch'ih on the lateral side of the occipital protuberance	Headache, torticollis, epistaxis, and asthma	As above
GB 20	Fêng-ch'ih 风池	* * *		
GB 21	Chien-chin 肩井	Midway between Ta-ch'ui and the acromion at the highest point of the shoulder	Pain in the shoulder and the back, torticollis, mastitis, and paralysis of the upper limbs	Perpendicularly 0.5 to 1.0 in. deep. Moxa heating for 10 to 30 min.

THE GALLBLADDER MERIDIAN OF FOOT—SHAOYANG (Cont.)

MERIDIAN NUMBER	NAME OF POINT	LOCATION	SPECIFIC INDICATIONS	TECHNIQUE
GB 22	Yüan-yeh 渊液	On the axillary line at the 4th intercostal space and 3 in. below the anterior axillary fold	Pleuritis, intercostal neuralgia, axillary lymphadenitis	Diagonally 0.5 to 1.0 in. deep. Moxa heating for 3 to 5 min.
GB 23	Che-chin 輒筋	At the 4th intercostal space, 1.0 in. anterior to Yüan-yeh	Emesis, asthma, and gastric hyperacidity	As above
GB 24	Jih-yüeh 日月	1 rib directly below Chi-mên at the 7th intercostal space	Hepatitis, gastralgia, cholecystitis, and hiccough	Diagonally 0.5 to 1.0 in. deep. Moxa heating for 10 to 20 min.
GB 25	Ching-mên 京门	At the tip of the 12th rib	Borborygmus, rib pain, and abdominal distention	Perpendicularly 0.3 to 0.5 in. deep. Moxa heating for 10 to 20 min.
GB 26	Tai-mo 带脉	* * *		
GB 27	Wu-shu 五枢	In front of the anterior superior iliac spine, 3.0 in. anterior and inferior to Tai-mo	Lower abdominal pain, lumbago, endometritis, and orchitis	Perpendicularly 1.0 to 1.5 in. deep. Moxa heating for 10 to 15 min.
GB 28	Wei-tao [illegible]	0.5 in. anterior and inferior to [illegible]	Endometritis, lower [illegible]	As above

GB 29	Chü-liao 居髎	* * *		
GB 30	Huan-t'iao 环跳	* * *		
GB 31	Fêng-shih 风市	* * *		
GB 32	Chung-tu 中渎	Lateral aspect of thigh, 2.0 in. below Fêng-shih	Hemiplegia and sciatica	Perpendicularly 1.5 to 2.5 in. deep. Moxa heating for 5 to 20 min.
GB 33	Ch'i-yang-kuan 膝阳关	In a depression above the lateral epicondyle of the femur, 3.0 in. above Yang-lin-ch'üan	Pain in the knee joint	Perpendicularly 0.5 to 0.8 in. deep
GB 34	Yang-lin-ch'üan 阳陵泉	* * *		
GB 35	Yang-chiao 阳交	7.0 in. above the tip of the external malleolus immediately anterior to the fibula	Sciatica, asthma, and pain in the lateral aspect of the leg	Perpendicularly 1.0 to 1.5 in. deep. Moxa heating for 5 to 25 min.
GB 36	Wai-chiu 外丘	1.0 in. directly posterior to Yang-chiao behind the fibula	Pain in the lateral aspect of the leg and gastrocnemius spasm	Perpendicularly 1.0 to 1.5 in. deep
GB 37	Kuang-ming 光明	2.0 in. directly distal to Yang-chiao	Eye diseases and pain in the lower limbs	Perpendicularly 0.5 to 1.5 in. deep. Moxa heating for 5 to 20 min.

THE GALLBLADDER MERIDIAN OF FOOT—SHAOYANG (Cont.)

MERIDIAN NUMBER	NAME OF POINT	LOCATION	SPECIFIC INDICATIONS	TECHNIQUE
GB 38	Yang-fu 阳輔	3.0 in. directly distal to Yang-chiao	Lumbago, arthritis of the knee joint, and malaise	As above
GB 39	Chüeh-ku 绝骨	* * *		
GB 40	Ch'iu-hsü 丘墟	* * *		
GB 41	Tsu-lin-ch'i 足临泣	* * *		
GB 42	Ti-wu-hui 地五会	Between the 4th and 5th metatarsals, 0.5 in. distal to Tsu-lin-ch'i	Mastitis, tinnitus, and pain in the axilla	Perpendicularly 0.3 to 0.5 in. deep
GB 43	Hsia-ch'i 侠溪	0.5 in. proximal to the margin of the web between the 4th and 5th toes	Headache, dizziness, deafness, chest pain, and intercostal neuralgia	Perpendicularly 0.3 to 0.5 in. deep. Moxa heating for 3 to 5 min.
GB 44	Tsu-chiao-yin 足窍阴	Immediately proximal to the lateral corner of the 4th toenail	Asthma, pleuritis, pharyngitis, and headache	Perpendicularly 0.1 to 0.2 in. deep. Moxa heating for 3 to 5 min.

Table 18

THE LIVER MERIDIAN OF FOOT—JUEYIN (Lv)

General indications: Chest congestion, emesis, lumbago, urinary retention, enuresis, hernia, and pain in the lower abdomen and along the course of this meridian

MERIDIAN NUMBER	NAME OF POINT	LOCATION	SPECIFIC INDICATIONS	TECHNIQUE
Lv 1	Ta-tun 大敦	Midway between the lateral corner of the 1st toenail and the interphalangeal joint	Enuresis, menorrhagia, and hernia	Diagonally 0.1 to 0.3 in. deep. Moxa heating for 5 to 7 min.
Lv 2	Hsing-chien 行间	0.5 in. proximal to the margin of the web between the 1st and 2d toes	Menstrual irregularity, urethritis, enuresis, hypertension, epilepsy, insomnia, and eye inflammation	Diagonally 0.3 to 0.5 in. deep. Moxa heating for 5 to 15 min.
Lv 3	T'ai-ch'ung 太冲	* * *		
Lv 4	Chung-fêng 中封	1.0 in. anterior to the medial malleolus, medial to the tendon of m. tibialis anticus	Lower abdominal pain, urinary retention, hernia, and pain of the penis	Perpendicularly 0.3 to 0.5 in. deep. Moxa heating for 5 to 15 min.
Lv 5	Li-kou 蠡沟	* * *		

THE LIVER MERIDIAN OF FOOT—JUEYIN (Cont.)

NUMBER MERIDIAN	NAME OF POINT	LOCATION	SPECIFIC INDICATIONS	TECHNIQUE
Lv 6	Chung-tu 中都	Posterior to the tibia, 7.0 in. above the tip of the medial malleolus	Menstrual irregularity, hernia, and pain of the joints of the lower extremities	Perpendicularly 0.5 to 1.5 in. deep. Moxa heating for 5 to 10 min.
Lv 7	Hsi-kuan 膝关	1.0 in. directly posterior to Yin-lin-ch'üan	Pain in the knee joint	Perpendicularly 1.0 to 1.5 in. deep. Moxa heating for 5 min.
Lv 8	Ch'u-ch'üan 曲泉	* * *		
Lv 9	Yin-pao 阴包	4 in. above the medial epicondyle of the femur between m. vastus medialis and m. sartorius	Lower abdominal pain, enuresis, lumbago, and menstrual irregularity	Perpendicularly 1.0 to 2.0 in. deep. Moxa heating for 5 to 10 min.
Lv 10	Tsu-wu-li 足五里	1.0 in. below Yin-lien, medial aspect of the thigh	Lower abdominal distention, urinary retention, enuresis, and scrotal eczema	As above
Lv 11	Yin-lien 阴廉	* * *		

Lv 12	Chi-mo 急脉	1.0 in. inferior and 2.5 in. lateral to the superior border of the symphysis pubis	Penile pain, uterine prolapse, pain in the lower abdomen and in the medial aspect of the thigh	Perpendicularly 0.5 to 1.0 in. deep, avoiding artery. Moxa heating for 5 to 15 min.
Lv 13	Chang-mên 章门	At the tip of the 11th rib	Diarrhea, abdominal distention, and pain in the costal region	Perpendicularly 0.5 to 0.8 in. deep. Moxa heating for 10 to 30 min.
Lv 14	Chi-mên 期门	At the 6th intercostal space directly below the nipple	Chest pain, pleuritis, hepatitis, and pain in the hypochondriac region	Diagonally 0.3 to 0.5 in. deep or 0.5 to 1.0 in. horizontally along the skin. Moxa heating for 5 to 15 min.

Table 19

THE GOVERNING VESSEL (DU, BACK MIDLINE) MERIDIAN (GV)

General indications: Fever, mental disorders, stiffness and pain of the spinal column, and opisthotonos

MERIDIAN NUMBER	NAME OF POINT	LOCATION	SPECIFIC INDICATIONS	TECHNIQUE
GV 1	Ch'ang-ch'iang 長强	* * *		
GV 2	Yao-yü 腰俞	At the junction between the sacrum and the coccyx	Lumbosacral pain, menstrual irregularity, impotence, prostatorrhea, enteritis and diarrhea	Diagonally 0.5 to 1.0 in. deep and cephalad
GV 3	Yao-yang-kuan 腰阳关	* * *		
GV 4	Ming-mên 命门	* * *		
GV 5	Hsuang-shu 悬枢	At the midline, between the 1st and the 2d vertebrae	Lumbago, dyspepsia, diarrhea, and enteritis	As above
GV 6	Chi-chung 脊中	At the midline, between the 11th and the 12th thoracic vertebrae	Epilepsy and bleeding hemorrhoids	Diagonally 0.5 to 1.0 in. deep and slightly cephalad. Moxa heat-

GV 7	Chung-shu 中枢	At the midline, between the 10th and the 11th thoracic vertebrae	Back pain, gastralgia, anorexia, and visual impairment	As above
GV 8	Chin-so 筋缩	At the midline between the 9th and the 10th thoracic vertebrae	Back pain, gastralgia, neurasthenia, epilepsy, and hysteria	As above
GV 9	Chih-yang 至阳	At the midline, between the 7th and the 8th thoracic vertebrae	Cough, dyspnea, jaundice, chest and back pain, and stiffness of the spinal column	As above
GV 10	Ling-tai 灵台	At the midline, between the 6th and 7th thoracic vertebrae	Asthma, bronchitis, lumbago, and gastralgia	As above
GV 11	Shên-tao 神道	At the midline, between the 5th and the 6th thoracic vertebrae	Poor memory, anxiety, stiffness of the back, and cough	Diagonally 0.5 to 1.0 in. deep and slightly cephalad. Moxa heating for 5 to 10 min.
GV 12	Shên-chu 身柱	At the midline, between the 3d and the 4th thoracic vertebrae	Cough, dyspnea, epilepsy, and stiffness and pain in the back	As above
GV 13	T'ao-tao 陶道	* * *		
GV 14	Ta-ch'ui 大椎	* * *		

THE GOVERNING VESSEL MERIDIAN (Cont.)

MERIDIAN NUMBER	NAME OF POINT	LOCATION	SPECIFIC INDICATIONS	TECHNIQUE
GV 15	Ya-mên 哑门	* * *		
GV 16	Fêng-fu 风府	At the midline, 1.0 in. above the hairline	Coryza, headache, mental disorders, and apoplexy	Perpendicularly 0.5 to 0.8 in. deep
GV 17	Nao-hu 脑户	1.5 in. directly above Fêng-fu	Stiffness and pain in the neck, headache, dizziness, and epilepsy	Diagonally 0.5 to 0.8 in. deep. Moxa heating for 2 to 3 min.
GV 18	Chiang-chien 强间	1.5 in. above Nao-hu midway between Fêng-fu and Pê-hui	Dizziness, headache, and emesis	Diagonally 0.5 to 0.8 in. deep. Moxa heating for 5 to 20 min.
GV 19	Hou-ting 后顶	1.5 in. directly above Chiang-chien	Vertigo, headache, and dizziness	As above
GV 20	Pê-hui 百会	* * *		
GV 21	Chien-ting 前顶	1.5 in. anterior to Pê-hui	Headache (vertex), dizziness, vertigo, facial swelling, and convulsions in children	As above

GV 22	Hsin-hui 囟会	3.0 in. anterior to Pê-hui	Headache, dizziness, vertigo, nasal obstruction, epistaxis, and convulsions in children	Diagonally 0.5 to 0.8 in. deep. Moxa heating for 3 to 5 min.
GV 23	Shang-hsin 上星	4.0 in. anterior to Pê-hui or 1.0 in. above the midpoint of the anterior hairline	Rhinitis, epistaxis, headache, eye diseases, and nasal obstruction	As above
GV 24	Shên-ting 神庭	0.5 in. above the hairline at the anterior midline	Headache (frontal), dizziness, vertigo, epilepsy, insomnia, rhinitis, and anxiety	As above
GV 25	Su-liao 素髎	At the tip of the nose	Epistaxis, rhinitis, nasal obstruction, and shock	Perpendicularly 0.2 to 0.3 in. deep
GV 26	Jen-chung 人中	* * *		
GV 27	Tui-tuan 兑端	At the junction of the philtrum and the upper lip directly below Jen-chung	Halitosis, toothache, and thrush	Diagonally 0.2 to 0.3 in. deep
GV 28	Yin-chiao 龈交	At the labial frenulum between the upper lip and the upper gum	Gingivitis and hemorrhoids	Diagonally upwards 0.1 to 0.2 in. deep, till blood is drawn

Table 20

THE CONCEPTION VESSEL (REN, FRONT MIDLINE) MERIDIAN (CV)

General indications: Hernia, leukorrhea, urogenital diseases, cough, and dyspnea

MERIDIAN NUMBER	NAME OF POINT	LOCATION	SPECIFIC INDICATIONS	TECHNIQUE
CV 1	Hui-yin 会阴	At the center of the perineum	Hemorrhoids, uterine prolapse, menstrual irregularity, pain of penis, and urethritis	Perpendicularly 0.5 to 1.0 in. deep. Moxa heating for 10 to 20 min.
CV 2	Ch'ü-ku 曲骨	* * *		
CV 3	Chung-chi 中极	* * *		
CV 4	Kuan-yüan 关元	* * *		
CV 5	Shih-mên 石门	At the midline, 2.0 in. below the umbilicus	Menstrual problems, leukorrhea, dysuria, abdominal distention, and edema	Perpendicularly 1.5 to 2.0 in. deep. Moxa heating for 20 to 30 min.
CV 6	Ch'i-hai 气海	* * *		

CV 7	Yin-chiao 阴交	At the midline, 1.0 in. below the umbilicus	Menstrual irregularity, endometritis, hernia, postpartum pain, pruritis vulvae, and urethritis	Perpendicularly 1.0 to 2.0 in. deep. Moxa heating for 10 to 20 min.
CV 8	Ch'i-chung 脐中	* * *		
CV 9	Shui-fên 水分	At the midline, 1.0 in. above the umbilicus	Diarrhea, dysuria,borborygmus, and edema	As above
CV 10	Hsia-kuan 下脘	At the midline, 2.0 in. above the umbilicus	Enteritis, gastralgia, gastroptosis, and dyspepsia	As above
CV 11	Chien-li 建里	At the midline, 3.0 in. above the umbilicus	Dyspepsia, peritonitis, gastralgia, emesis, and edema	As above
CV 12	Chung-kuan 中脘	* * *		
CV 13	Shang-kuan 上脘	At the midline, 5.0 in. above the umbilicus	Abdominal distention, gastritis, gastric ulcer, emesis, and hiccough	Perpendicularly 1.0 to 2.0 in. deep. Moxa heating for 10 to 20 min.
CV 14	Chü-chieh 巨闕	At the midline, 6.0 in. above the umbilicus	Emesis, gastralgia, anxiety, and palpitation	Diagonally 1.0 in. deep and caudad. Moxa heating for 10 to 20 min.

THE CONCEPTION VESSEL MERIDIAN (Cont.)

MERIDIAN NUMBER	NAME OF POINT	LOCATION	SPECIFIC INDICATIONS	TECHNIQUE
CV 15	Chiu-wei 鸠尾	* * *		
CV 16	Chung-ting 中庭	At the midline, 1.6 in. directly below Tan-chung	Emesis, cough, asthma, and regurgitation	Diagonally 0.3 to 0.5 in. deep. Moxa heating for 5 to 20 min.
CV 17	Tan-chung 膻中	* * *		
CV 18	Yü-tang 玉堂	At the midline, 1.6 in. above Tan-chung, level with the 3d intercostal space	Emesis, asthma, pleuritis, and bronchitis	As above
CV 19	Tsu-kung 紫宫	At the midline level with the 2d intercostal space, 3.2 in. above Tan-chung	Pleuritis and bronchitis	As above
CV 20	Hua-kai 华盖	At the junction of the sternal manubrium and body at the midline	Asthma, cough, chest pain, and pharyngitis	As above
CV 21	Hsüan-chi 璇璣	* * *		
CV 22	T'ien-t'u	* * *		

CV 23	Lien ch'üan 廉泉	* * *		
CV 24	Ch'êng-chiang 承浆	* * *		

L = *The Lung Meridian of Hand—Taiyin*
LI = *The Large Intestine Meridian of Hand—Yangming*
S = *The Stomach Meridian of Foot—Yangming*
Sp = *The Spleen Meridian of Foot—Taiyin*
H = *The Heart Meridian of Hand—Shaoyin*
SI = *The Small Intestine Meridian of Hand—Taiyang*
B1 = *The Bladder Meridian of Foot—Taiyang*
K = *The Kidney Meridian of Foot—Shaoyin*
CS = *The Circulation-Sex Meridian of Hand—Jueyin*
T = *The Triple Warmer Meridian of Hand—Shayang*
GB = *The Gallbladder Meridian of Foot—Shaoyang*
Lv = *The Liver Meridian of Foot—Jueyin*
GV = *The Governing Vessel Meridian*
CV = *The Conception Vessel Meridian*

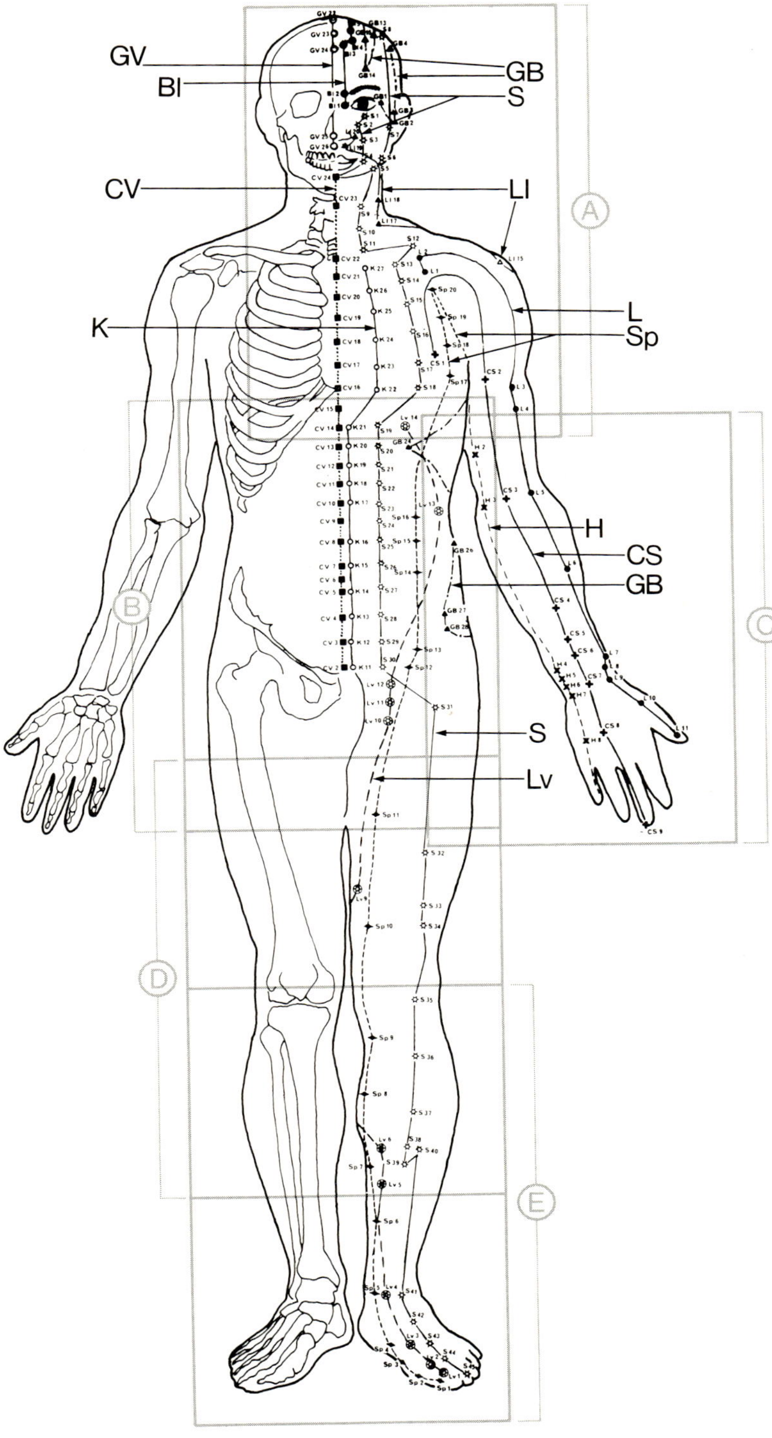

Fig. 49 Meridian distribution of acupuncture points (front view)

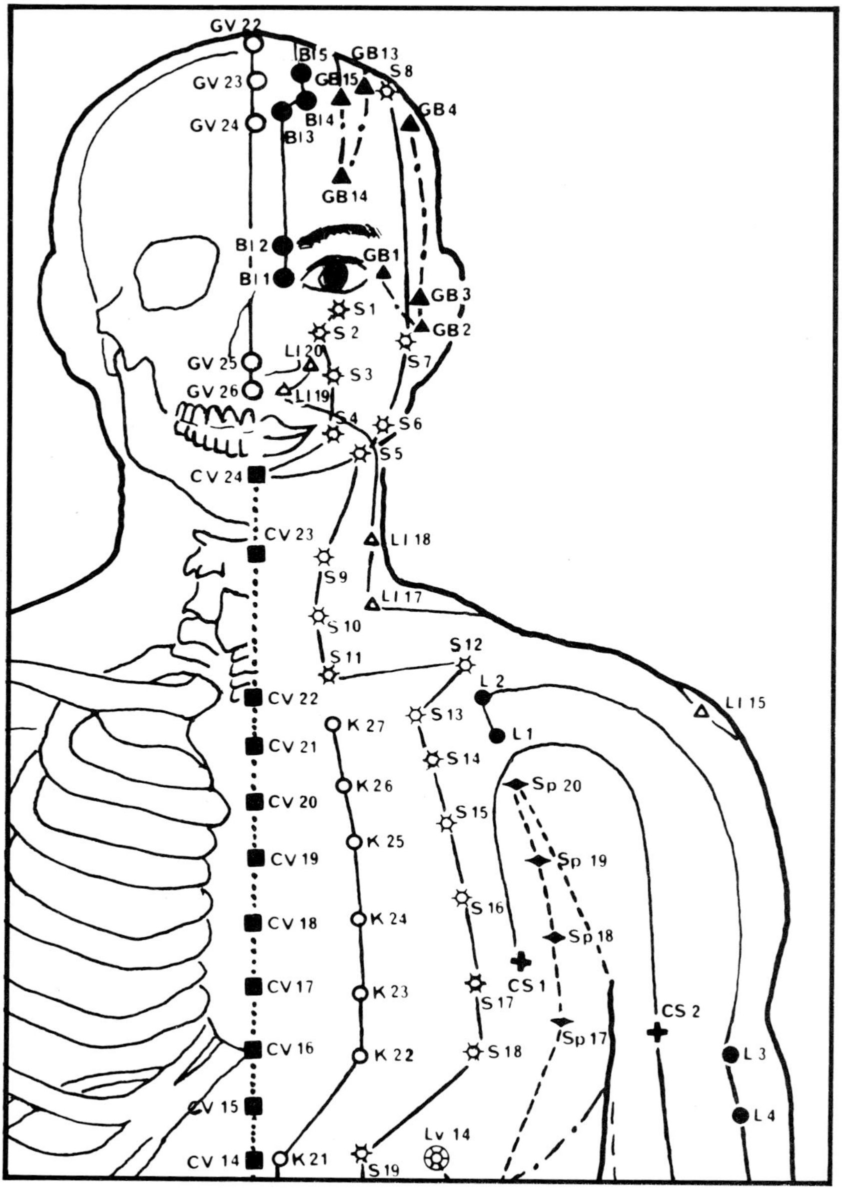

Fig. 49 (cont.)
Front view, section A

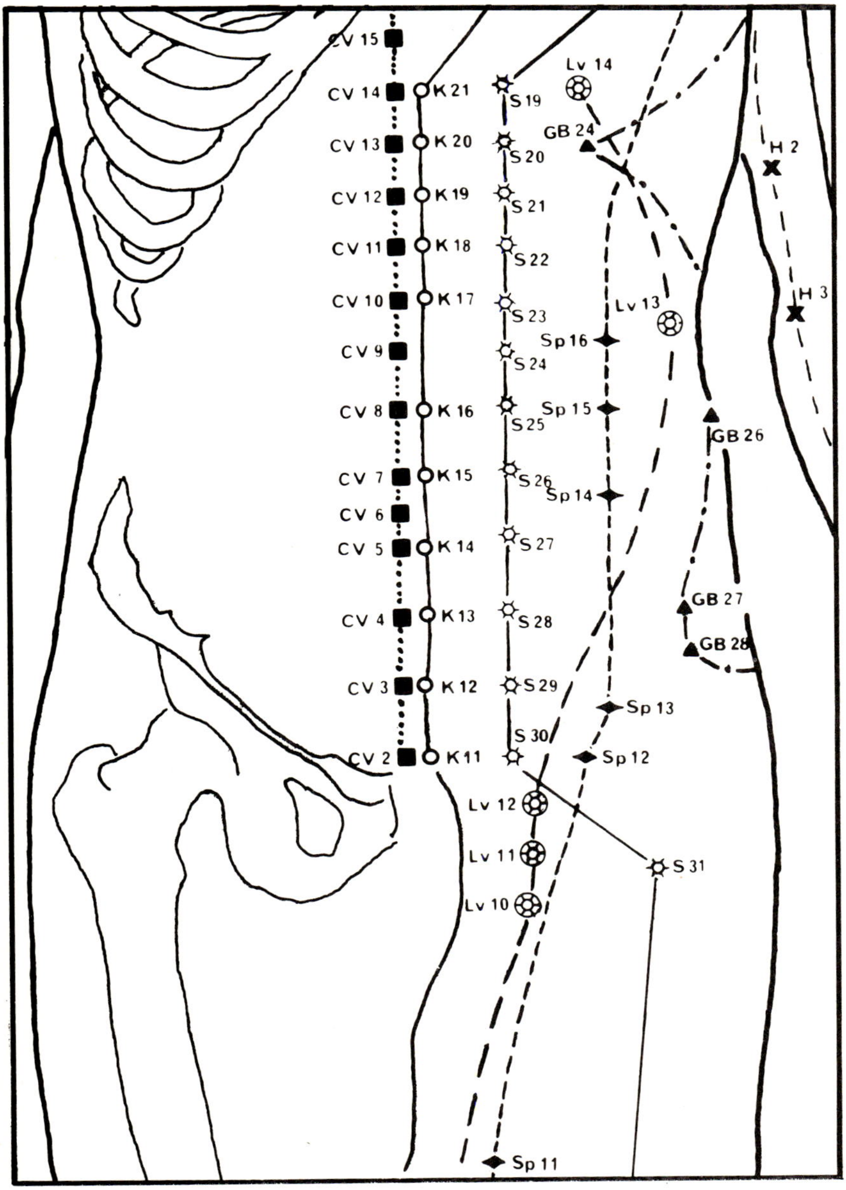

Fig. 49 (cont.)
Front view, section B

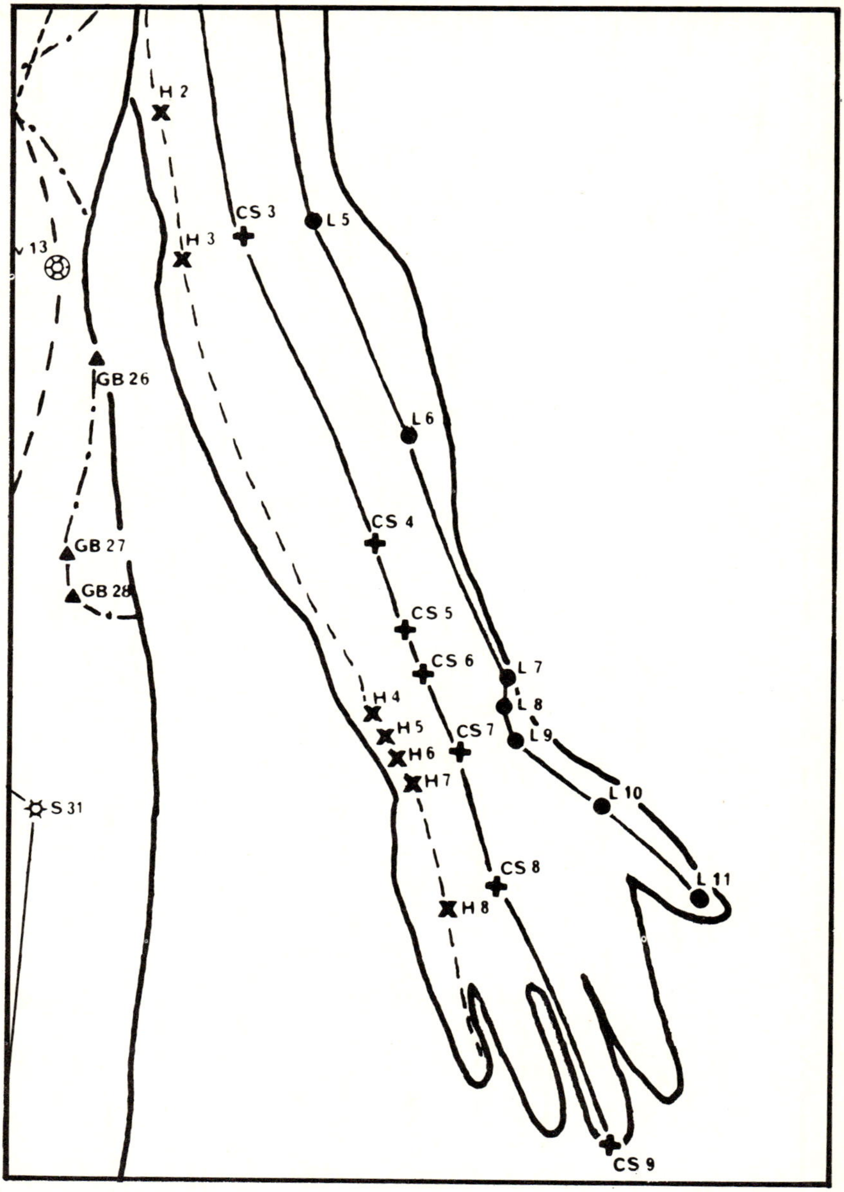

Fig. 49 (cont.)
Front view, section C

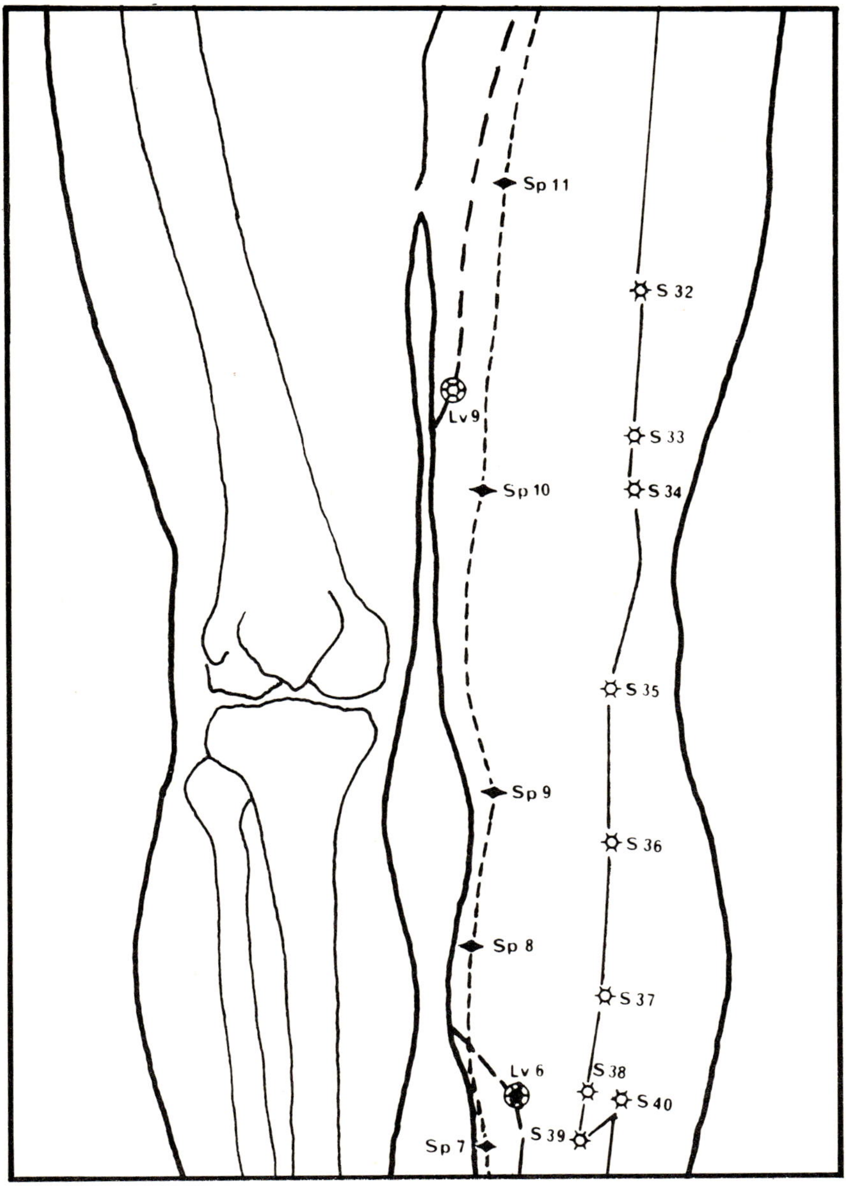

Fig. 49 (cont.)
Front view, section D

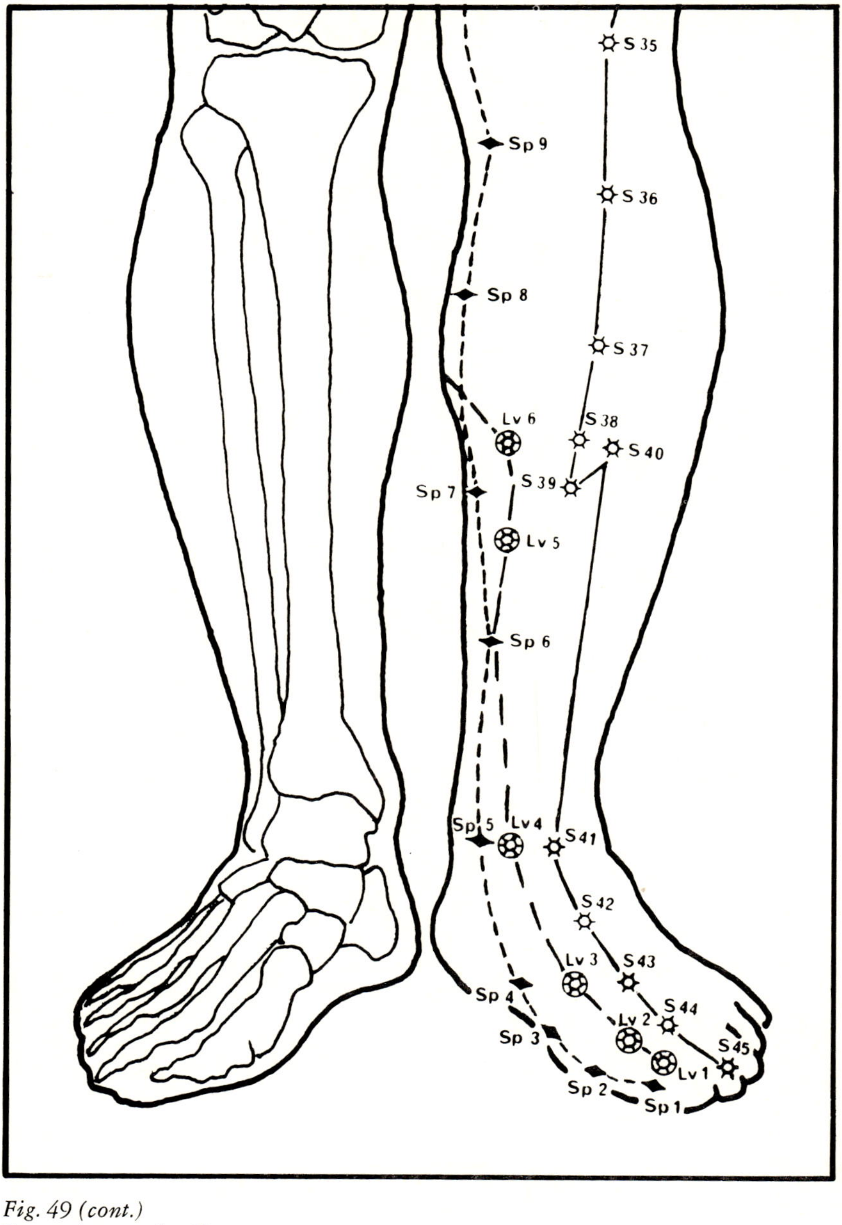

Fig. 49 (cont.)
Front view, section E

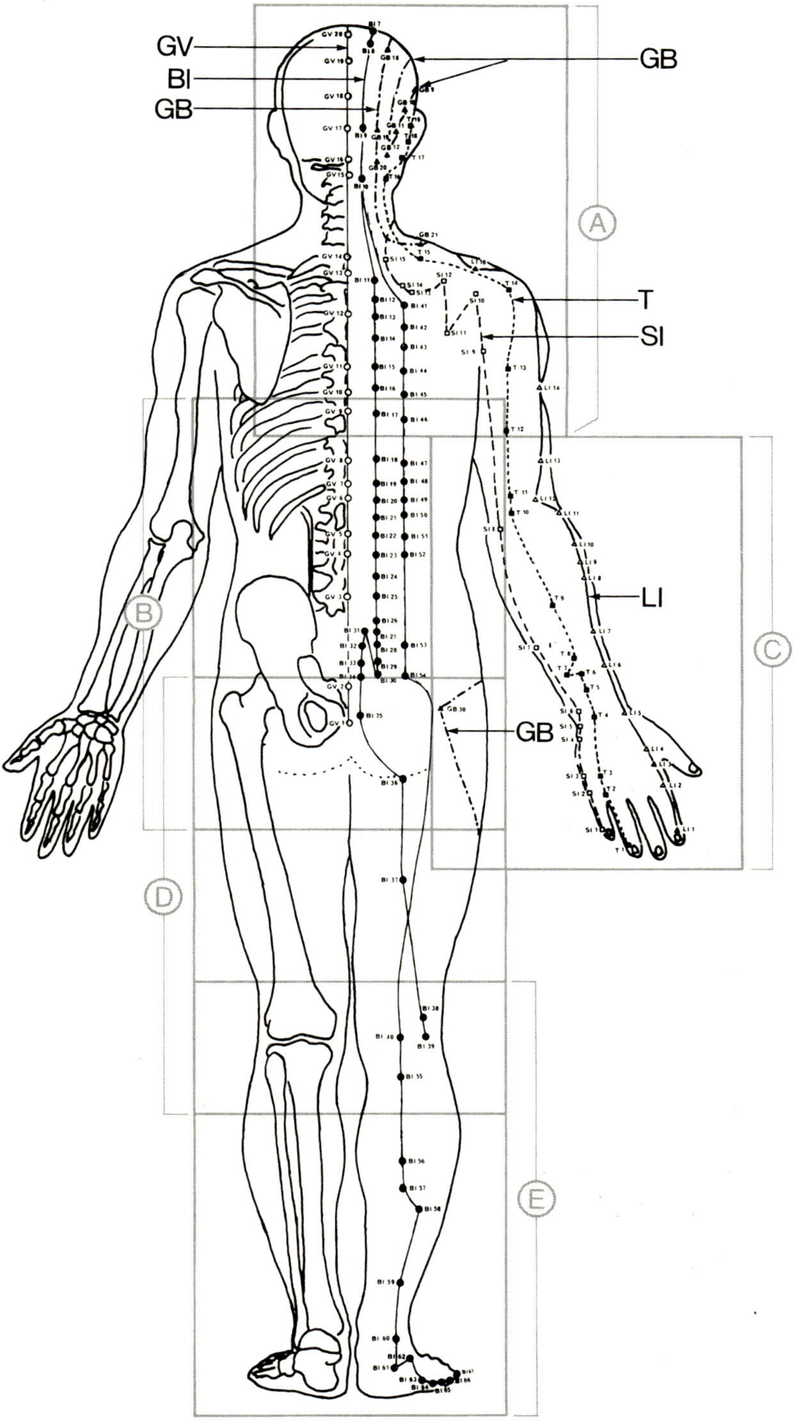

Fig. 50 Meridian distribution of acupuncture points (back view)

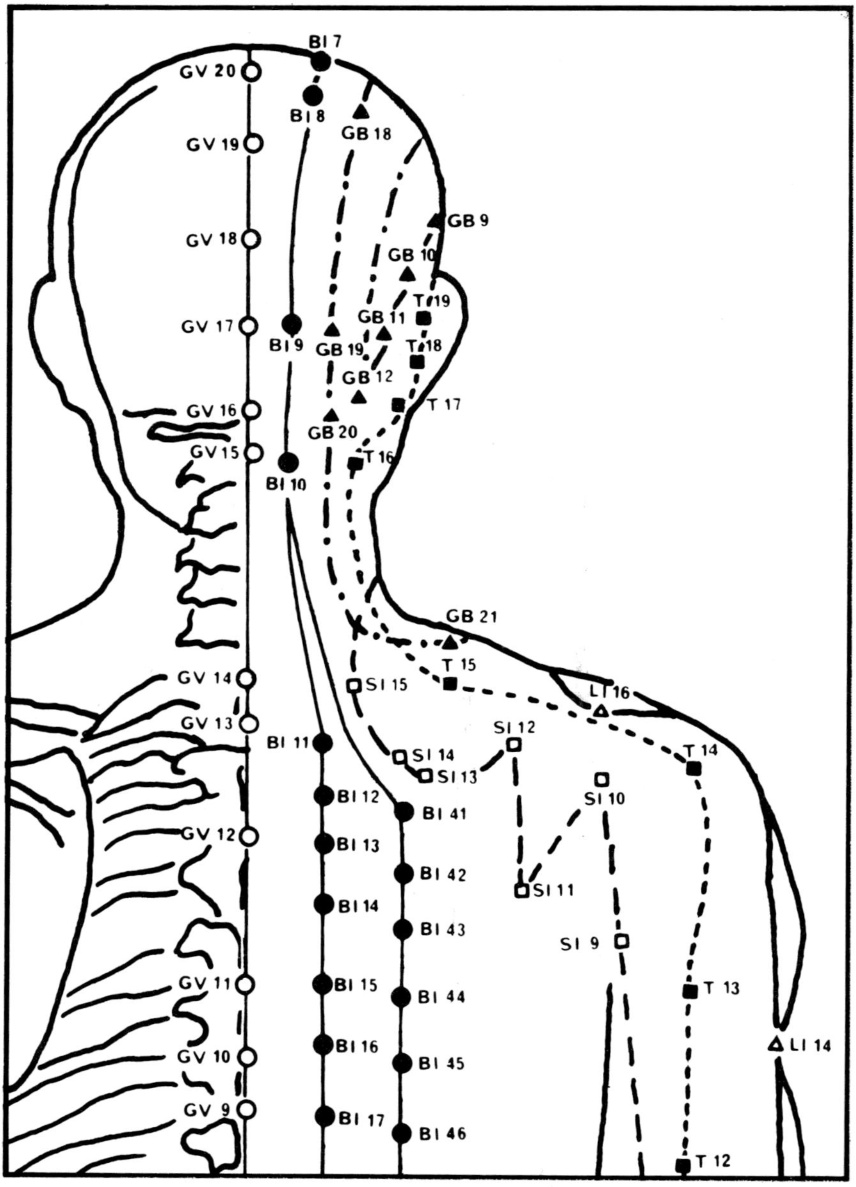

Fig. 50 (cont.)
Back view, section A

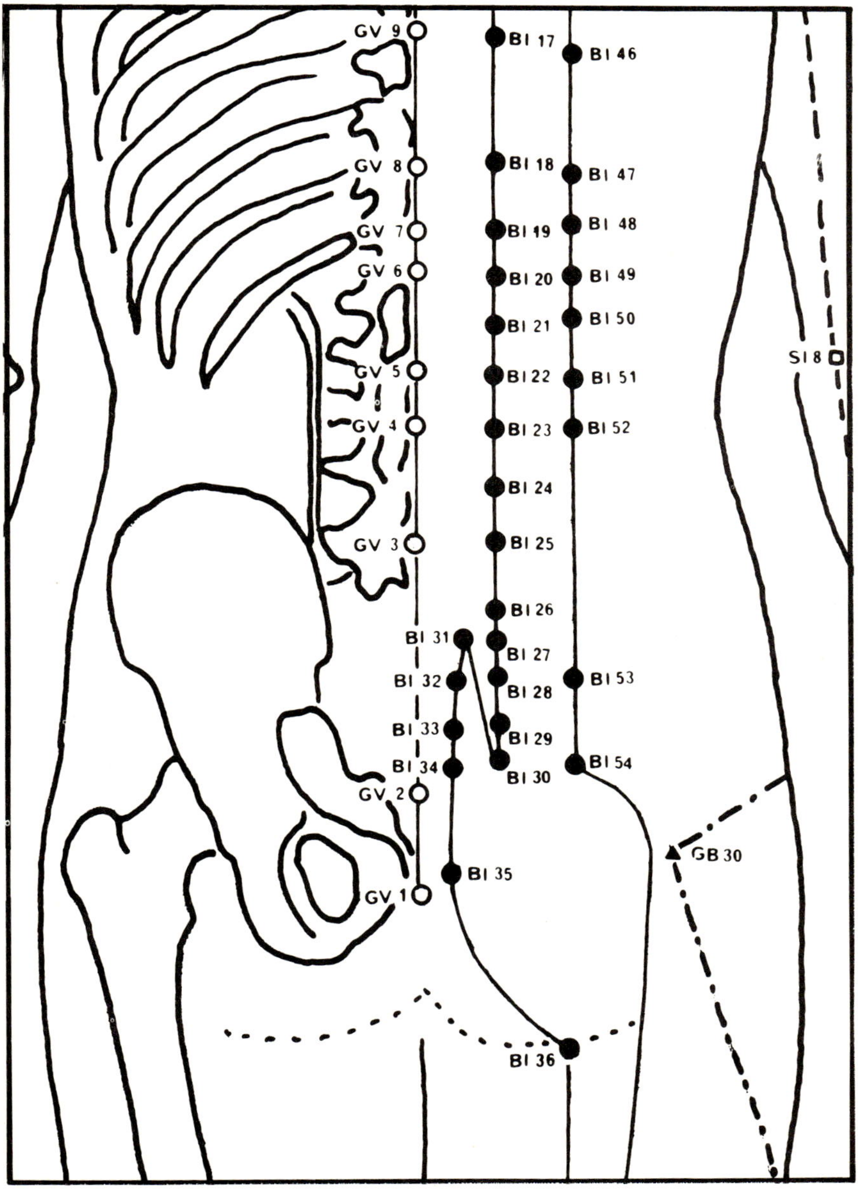

Fig. 50 (cont.)
Back view, section B

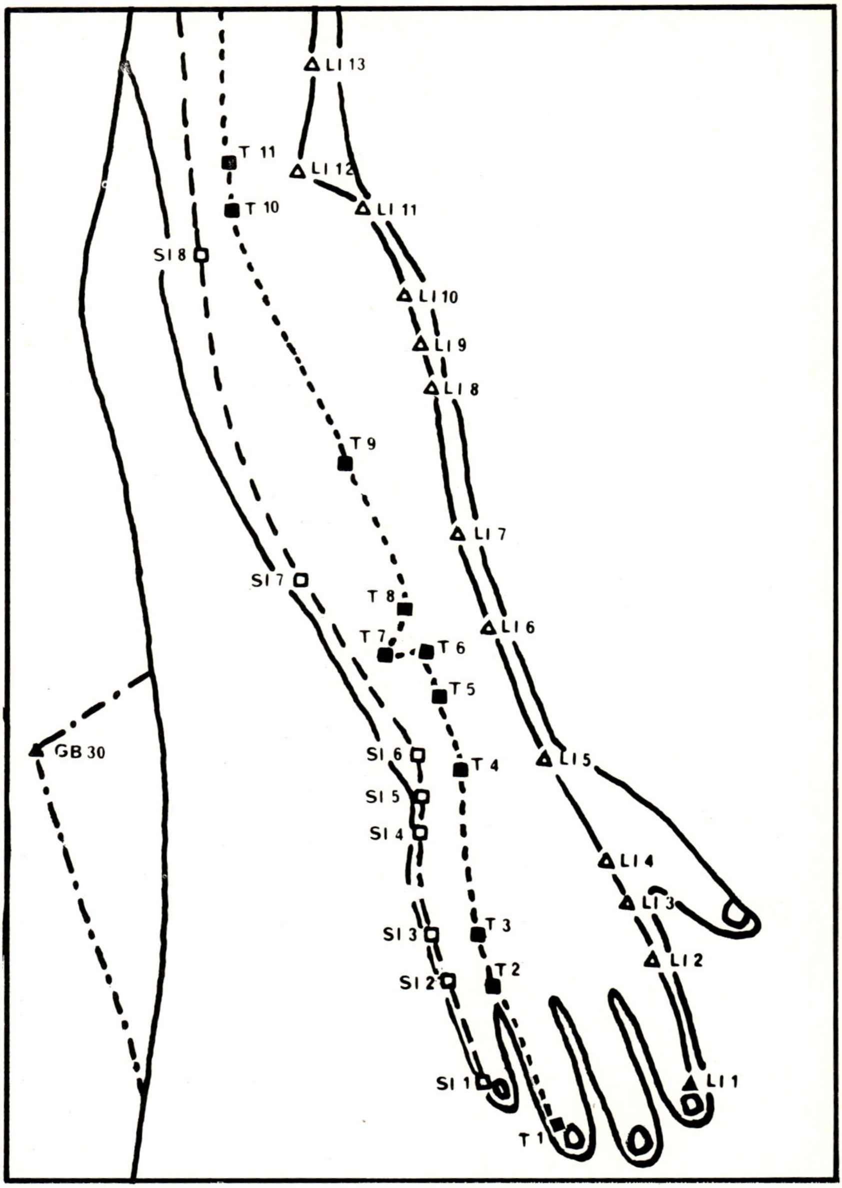

Fig. 50 (cont.)
Back view, section C

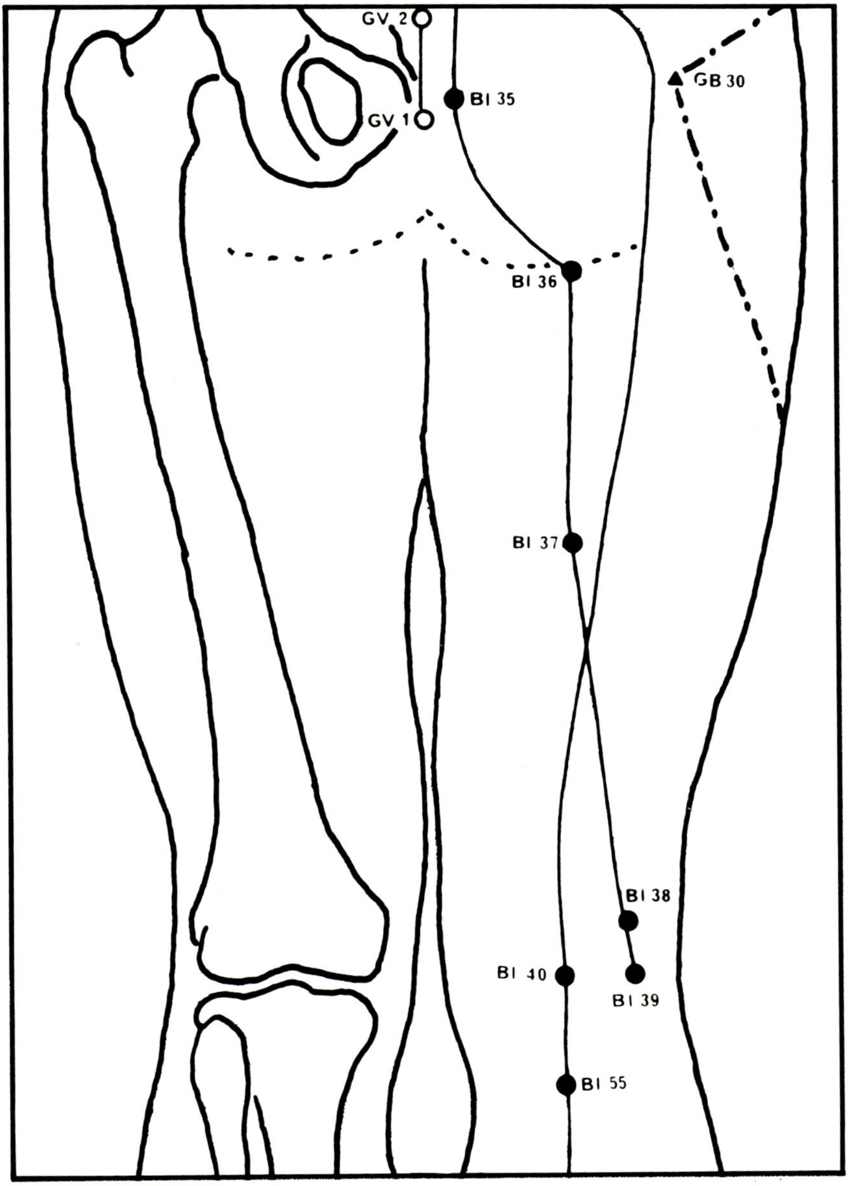

Fig. 50 (cont.)
Back view, section D

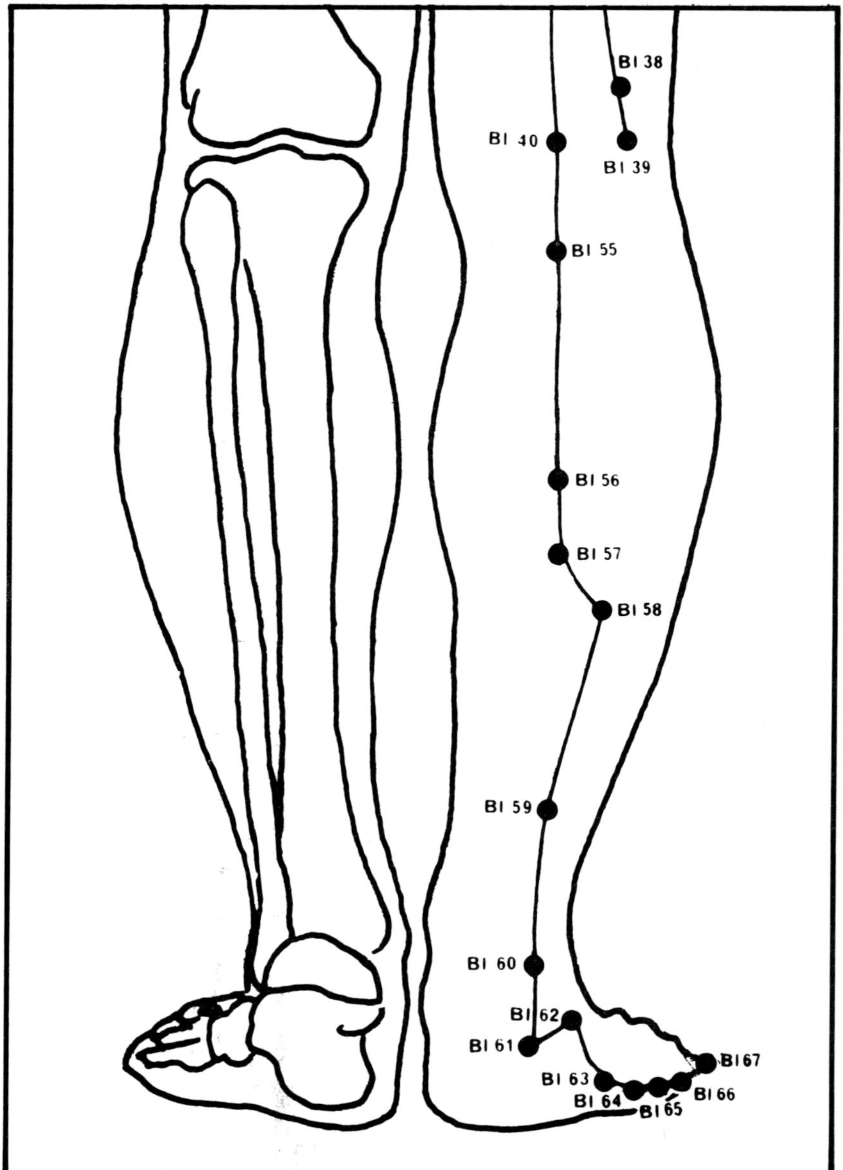

Fig. 50 (cont.)
Back view, section E

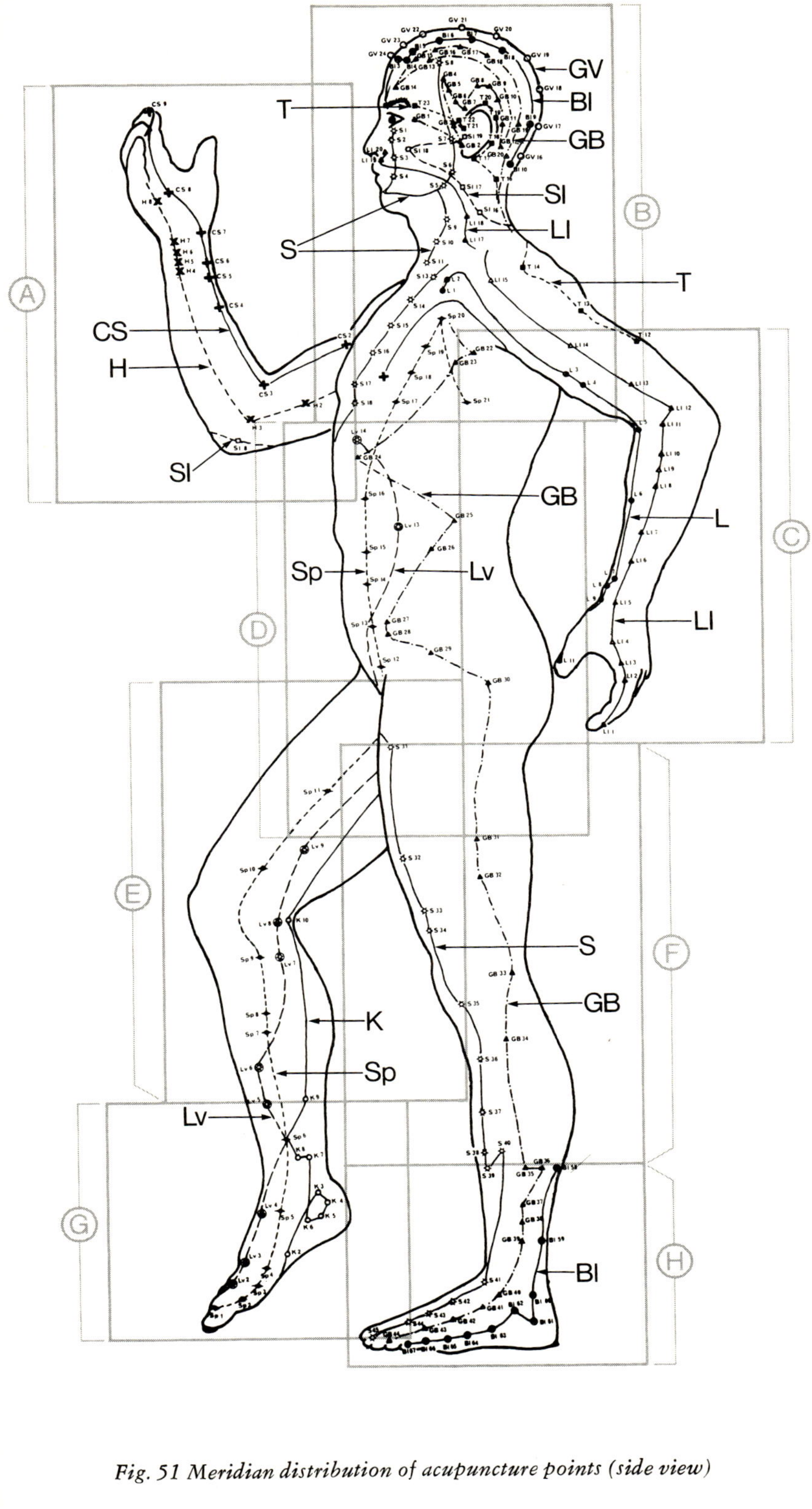

Fig. 51 Meridian distribution of acupuncture points (side view)

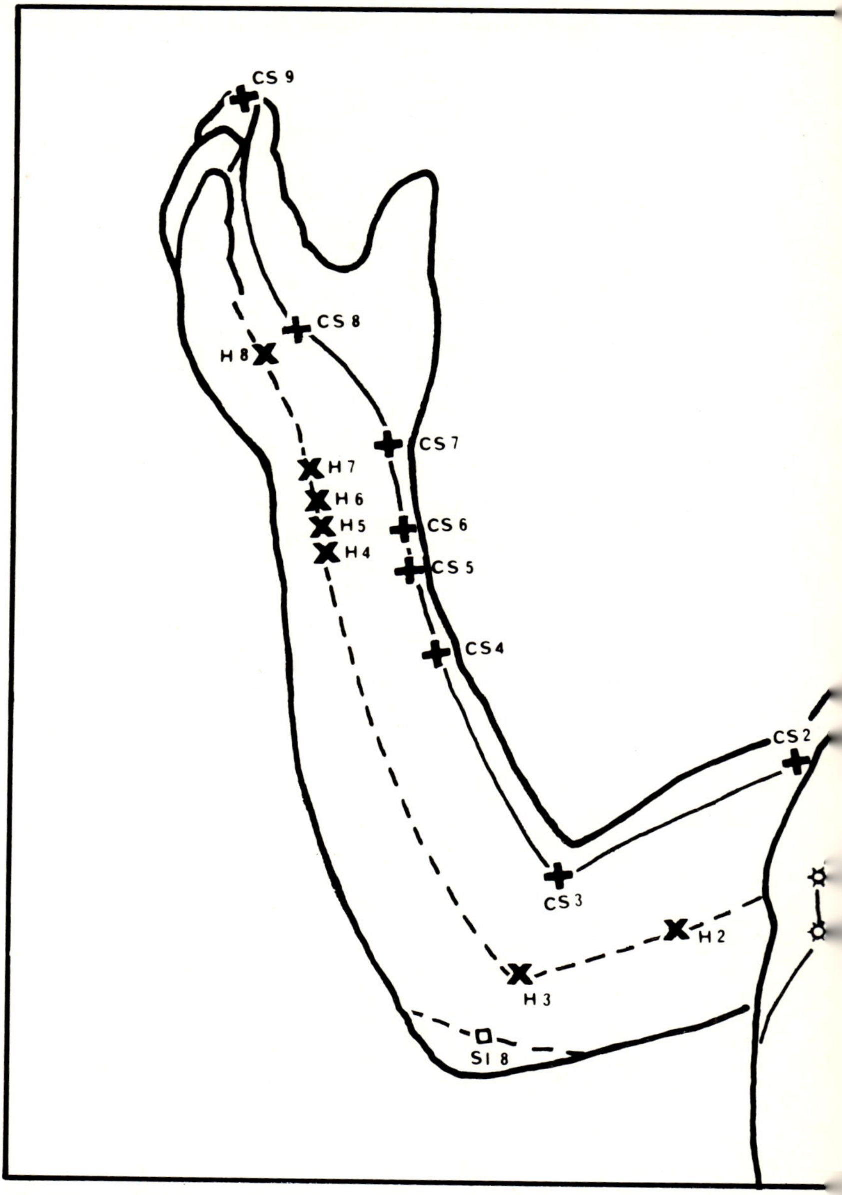

Fig. 51 (cont.)
Side view, section A

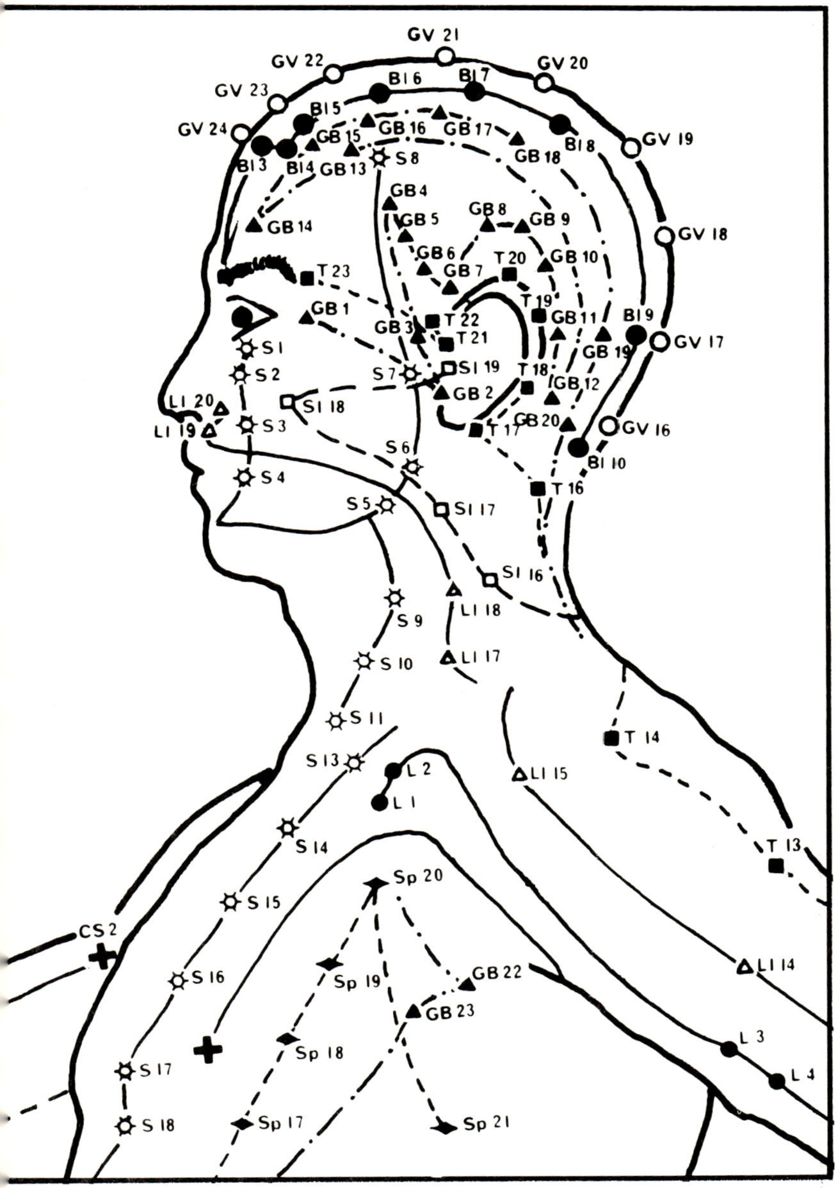

Fig. 51 (cont.)
Side view, section B

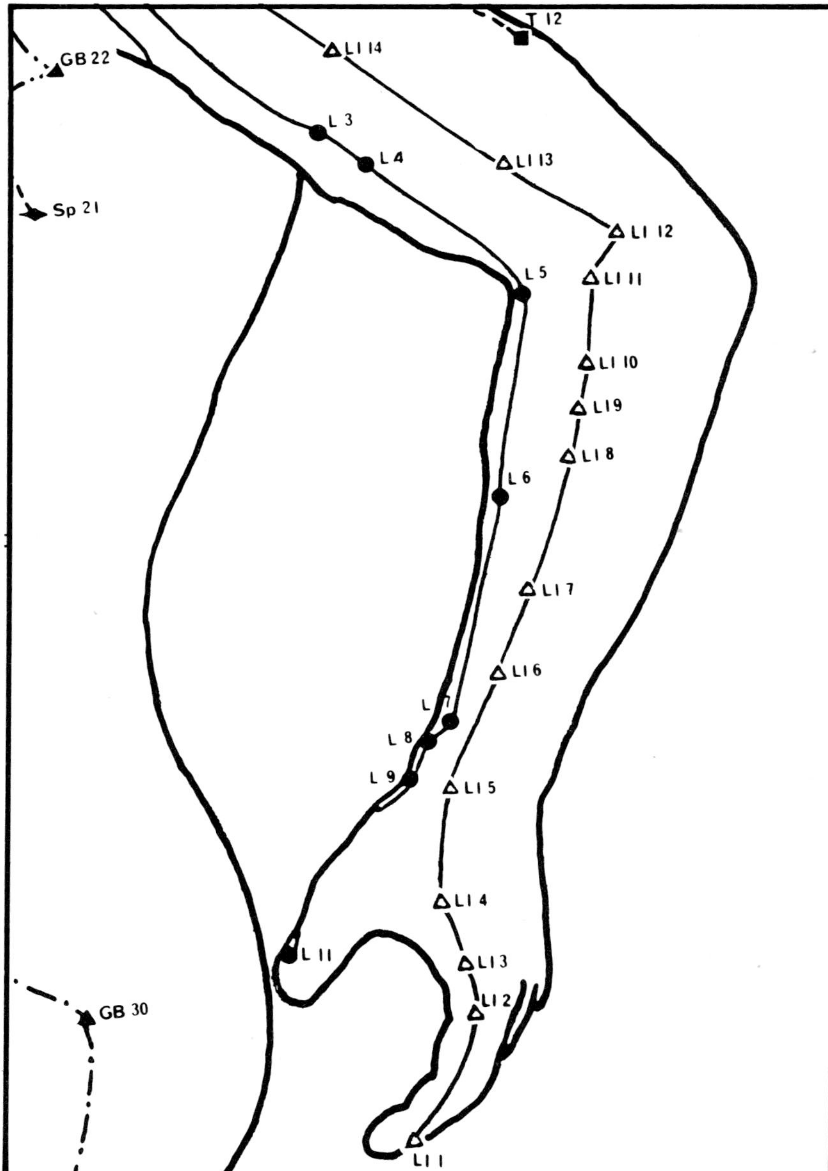

Fig. 51 (cont.)
Side view, section C

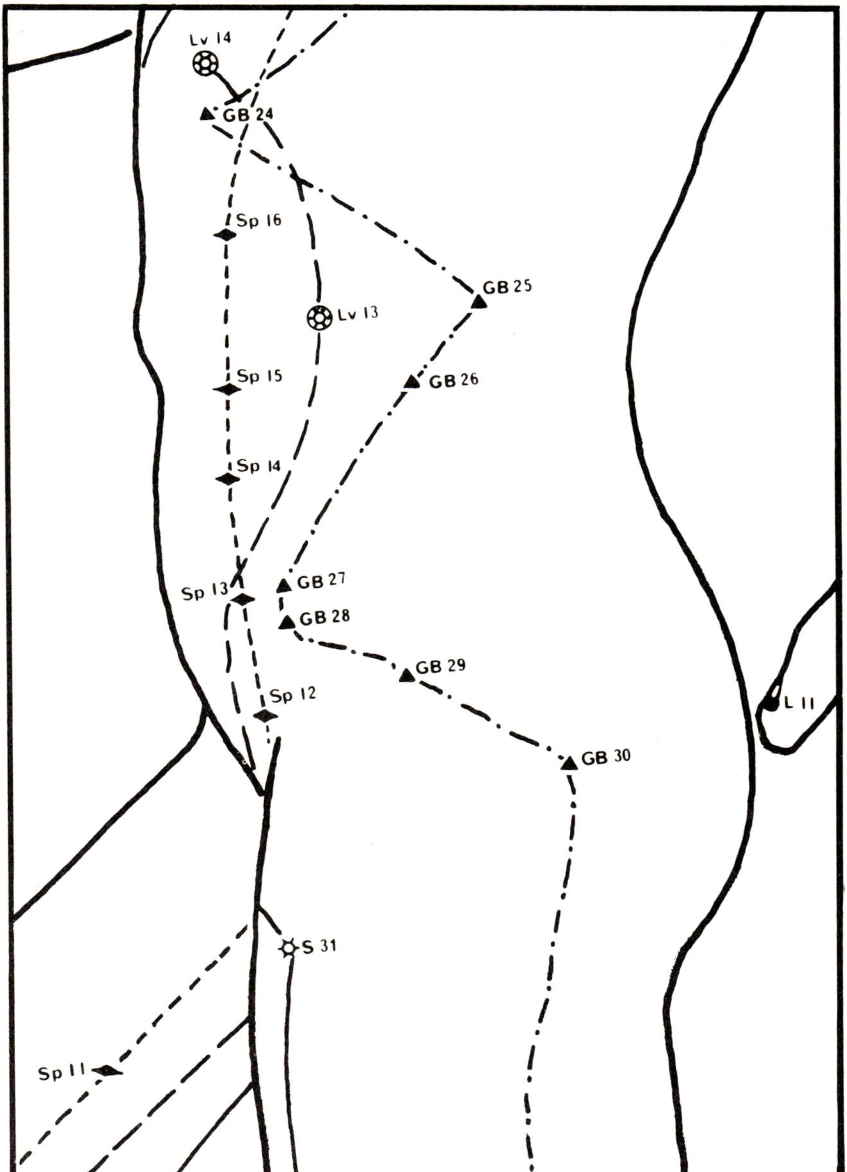

Fig. 51 (cont.)
Side view, section D

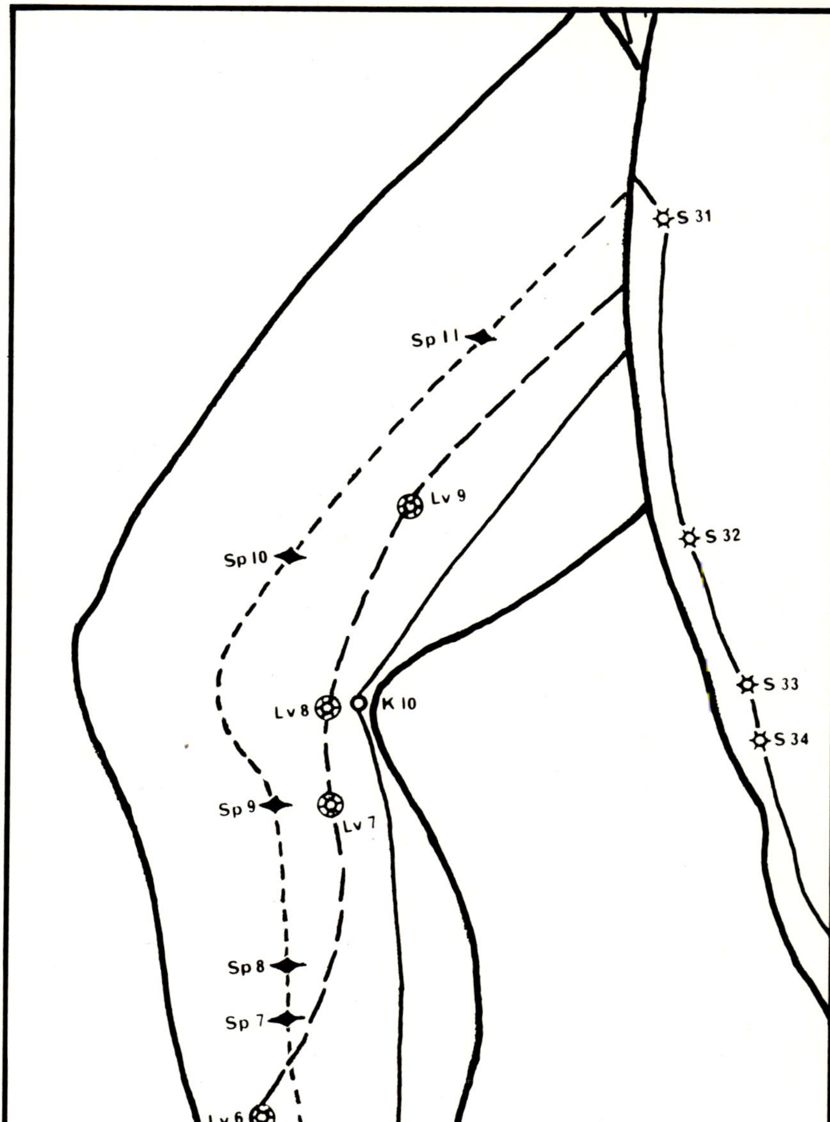

Fig. 51 (cont.)
Side view, section E

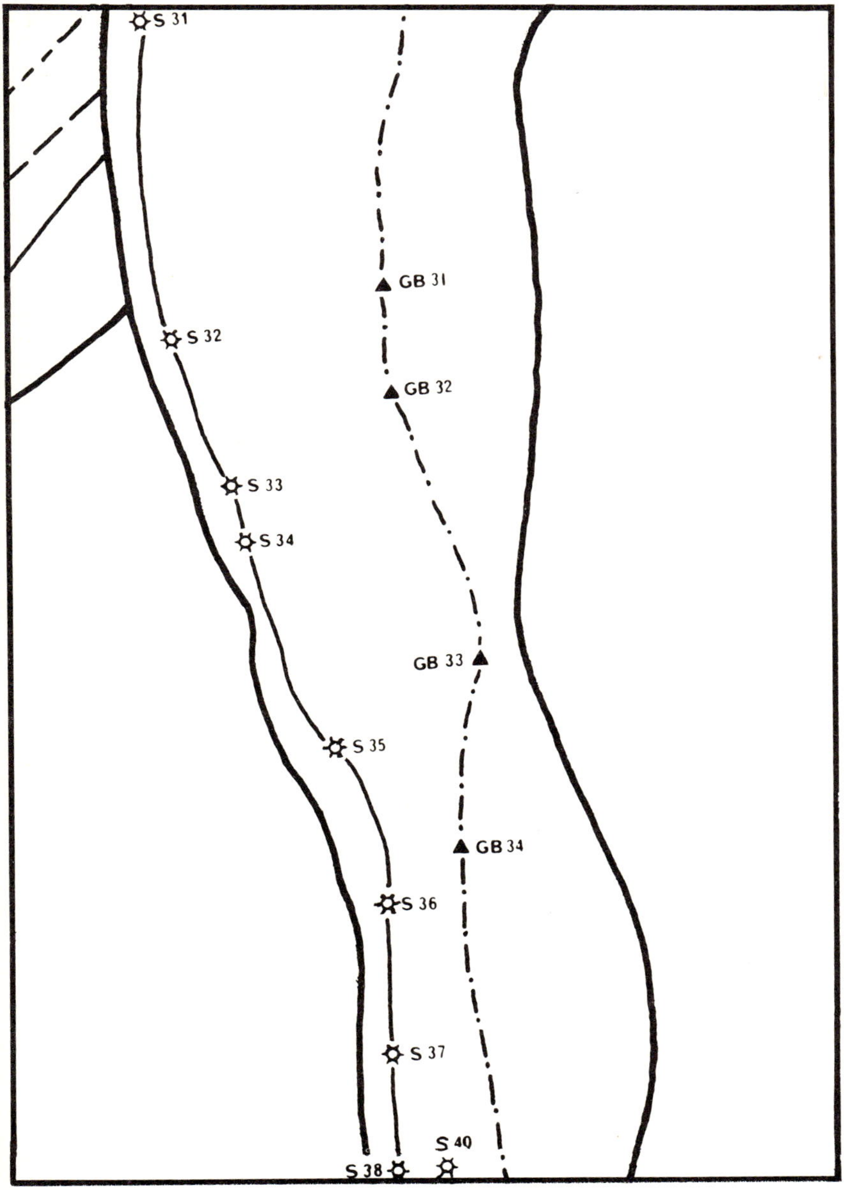

Fig. 51 (cont.)
Side view, section F

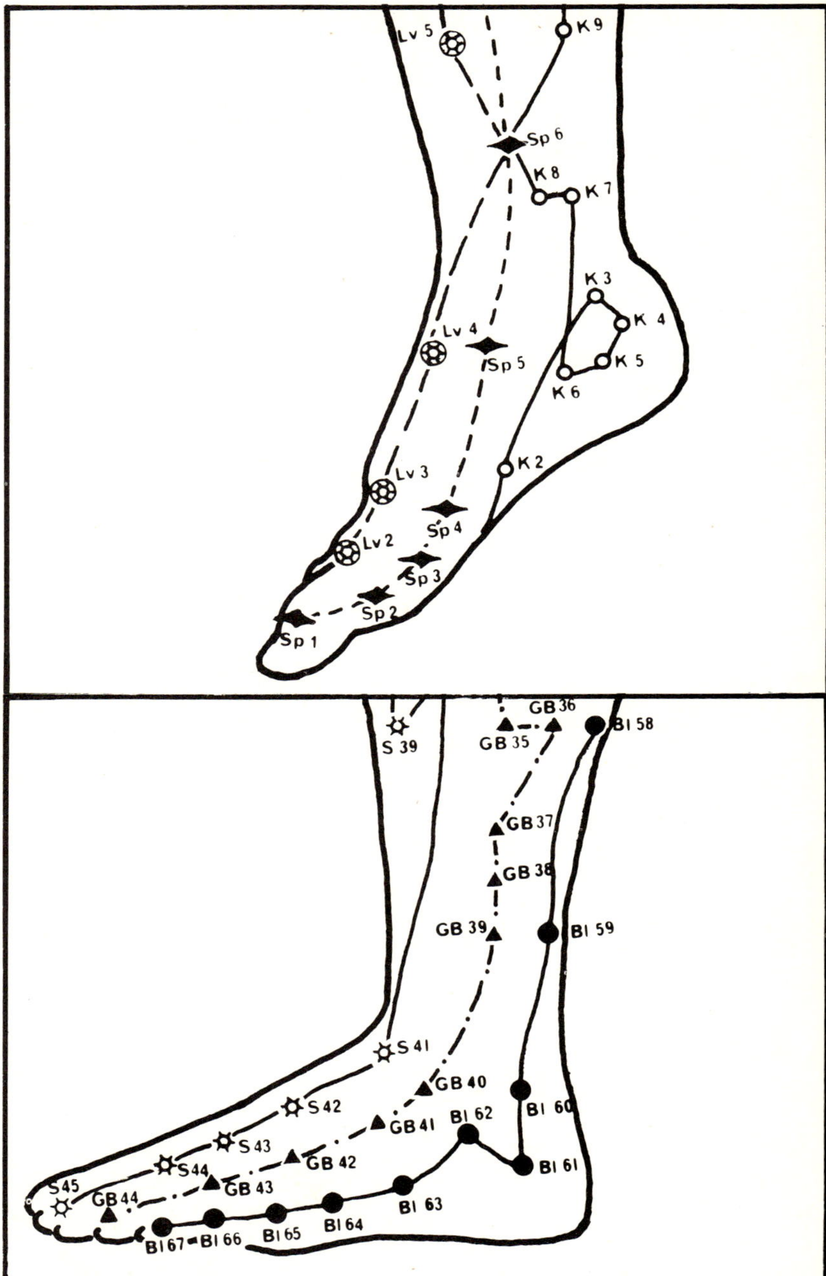

Fig. 51 (cont.)
Side view, sections G and H

DISEASES AND SYMPTOMS AMENABLE TO ACUPUNCTURE THERAPY

4 DISEASES AND SYMPTOMS AMENABLE TO ACUPUNCTURE THERAPY

SELECTION OF POINTS FOR TREATMENT

In acupuncture therapy, treatment of a disease or symptom is accomplished by stimulation of a properly selected single acupuncture point or of a combination of several points. The number of main points or supplemental points to be used for a specific complaint varies, but in general is governed by the response to therapy. Certain diseases may improve dramatically by stimulation of just one or two of the main points specific for the disease, while others may require additional main points as well as supplemental points. In instituting treatment, it is customary to use the specific main points initially and, judging from the response, resort to supplemental points when necessary.

Acupuncture points are selected from one or a combination of the following categories of points:

1. Points situated in the proximity of the anatomical location of the disease or symptom. For example, the points for frontal headache, Yang-pê and Yin-t'ang; for temporal headache, T'ai-yang and Shuai-ku; and for goiter, Ch'i-yin.
2. Points situated at a distant site but which are held to exert a regulatory effect over specific diseased organs or the source of a symptom. These are exemplified by the specific points Lan-wei-hsüeh for appendicitis, Tan-nang-hsüeh and Nei-kuan for dis-

eases of the gallbladder and bile ducts, and Tsu-san-li, a main point for the amelioration of gastralgia and ileus.

3. Points selected for their efficacy in relieving specific symptoms. Noteworthy amongst these are the points Jen-chung and Shao-shang for syncope, Ta-ch'ui, Ch'ü-ch'ih and Ho-ku for fever, Nei-kuan and Tsu-san-li for nausea and emesis.
4. Pressure points which occur during the course of a disease. These points are usually found in the vicinity of the affected area, but they may also be located at a distant site, as in the case of the specific point for the treatment of appendicitis, Lan-wei-hsüeh, and also a main point for the treatment of diseases of the gall-bladder and bile ducts, Tan-nang-hsüeh. Digital pressure on these pressure points will yield point tenderness prior to treatment of the condition.
5. Ear points. These points may be employed to complement the common acupuncture points.

Table 21

EXAMPLES OF COMBINATIONS OF LOCAL AND DISTANT ACUPUNCTURE POINTS IN THE TREATMENT OF DISEASES

DISEASE LOCATION		LOCAL ACUPUNCTURE POINTS	DISTANT ACUPUNCTURE POINTS
Head	Frontal	Yin-t'ang, Yang-pe	Ho-ku, Nei-t'ing
	Temporal	T'ai-yang, Shuai-ku	Chung-chu, Tsu-lin-ch'i
	Occipital	Fêng-ch'ih, T'ien-chu	Hou-ch'i, Shuai-ku
	Vertex	Pê-hui	T'ai-ch'ung
Eye		Ching-ming, Ch'êng-ch'i, Fêng-ch'ih	Ho-ku
Nose		Yin-t'ang, Yin-hsiang	Ho-ku
Mouth and teeth		Chia-ch'ê, Hsia-kuan, Ti-ts'ang	Ho-ku
Tongue		Lien-ch'üan,	Ho-ku
Throat		T'ien-yung	Ho-ku, Shao-shang
Trachea		T'ien-t'u	Lieh-ch'üeh
Lung		Fei-yü, Tan-chung, T'ien-t'u	Lieh-ch'üeh, Ch'ih-che
Heart		Hsin-yü, Tan-chung	Nei-kuan, Shên-mên, Chien-shih
Stomach		Wei-yü, Chung-kuan	Nei-kuan, Tsu-san-li
Liver		Kan-yü	T'ai-ch'ung
Gallbladder		Tan-yü	Tan-nang-hsüeh, Yang-lin-ch'üan
Intestines		Ta-ch'ang-yü, Hsiao-ch'ang-yü, T'ien-shu, Kuan-yüan	Shang-chü-hsü, Tsu-san-li
Kidney		Shêng-yü, Chih-shih	T'ai-ch'i
Bladder		Ts'ŭ-liao, Chung-chi	San-yin-chiao
Reproductive system		Chung-chi, Kuan-yüan, Tzŭ-kung	San-yin-chiao
Anus		Ch'ang-ch'iang, Chih-pien	Ch'êng-san
Upper extremity		Chien-yü, Ch'ü-ch'ih, Ho-ku	
Lower extremity		Huan-t'iao, Wei-chung, Yang-lin-ch'üan, Chüeh-ku	

Table 22

ACUPUNCTURE POINTS FOR TREATMENT OF SPECIFIC SYMPTOMS

SYMPTOMS	ACUPUNCTURE POINTS (EXAMPLES)
Fever	Ta-ch'ui, Ch'ü-ch'ih, Ho-ku
Syncope	Jen-chung, Shih-hsüan
Shock	Tsu-san-li, Pê-hui, Kuan-yüan, Ch'i-chung
Excessive perspiration	Ho-ku, Fu-liu
Insomnia	Shên-mên, San-yin-chiao, T'ai-ch'i
Hoarseness	Ho-ku, Chien-shih, Fuh-t'u
Diarrhea	Shang-chü-hsü, T'ien-shu
Dysphagia	T'ien-t'u, Nei-kuan, Ho-ku, Fuh-t'u
Excessive salivation	Jen-chung, Chia-ch'ê, Ho-ku
Cough	T'ien-t'u, Lieh-ch'üeh
Heart palpitation	Nei-kuan, Hsi-mên
Chest pain	Tan-chung, Nei-kuan
Vomiting	Nei-kuan, Tsu-san-li
Dyspepsia	Tsu-san-li, Kung-sun
Dysarthria	Ya-mên, Lien-ch'üan, Ho-ku
Abdominal distention	T'ien-shu, Ch'i-hai, Nei-kuan, Tsu-san-li
Urinary retention	San-yin-chiao, Yin-lin-ch'üan
Incontinence of urine	Ch'ü-ku, San-yin-chiao
Impotence	Kuan-yüan, San-yin-chiao
Constipation	T'ien-shu, Chih-kou
Rectal prolapse	Ch'ang-ch'iang, Ch'êng-san
Gastrocnemius spasm	Ch'êng-san
Pruritus	Ch'ü-ch'ih, Hsüeh-hai
Chronic fatigue	Kuan-yüan, Tsu-san-li

LIST OF DISEASES AND SYMPTOMS

Enumerated here is a list of diseases and symptoms representative of ailments that are purported to respond well to acupuncture therapy. This list is selective and by no means complete. For each of the conditions mentioned, the common acupuncture points recommended for its treatment are listed. Also included are the ear points, whose usage, however, is optional.

SYNCOPE

Main points. Jen-chung (HN–18), Shao-shang (UE–23). Strong stimulation is recommended. The patient should be in Trendelenberg position.
Moxa heating. Pê-hui (HN–1).

MALARIA

Main points. Ta-ch'ui (B–1), T'ao-tao (B–2), Nei-kuan (UE–26), Chien-shih (UE–25).
Supplemental points. Ch'ü-ch'ih (UE–7), Tsu-san-li (LE–10), Yang-lin-ch'üan (LE–15).

Treatment should be instituted 2 to 3 hours before each episode of chills occurs. Strong stimulation for a brief period or intermittent twirling for 15 to 30 minutes is recommended.

UPPER RESPIRATORY INFECTIONS

Main points. Fêng-ch'ih (HN–25), Ho-ku (UE–12).
Supplemental points. Yin-hsiang (HN–17), T'ai-yang (HN–3), Fêng-mên (B–4), Ta-ch'ui (B–1).

Asthma

Main points. Ch'uan-hsi (B–3), T'ien-t'u (CA–1), Hsüan-chi (CA–2), Tan-chung (CA–3), Chiai-ch'uan (B–26).
Supplemental points. Ho-ku (UE–12), Tsu-san-li (LE–10).

Between the acute asthmatic episodes, any 2 to 4 of the main points along with the supplemental points may be used for treatment of the disease. Treatment is performed once daily and for a period of 7 to 10 days. For an acute attack, the main points Hsüan-chi and Tan-chung are used. Continuous twirling of the inserted needle for 2 to 5 minutes is recommended. If relief is not forthcoming, the main point Chiai-ch'uan is used in addition. This point is stimulated for 10 to 20 minutes.

Ear points. The point is located at the specific site for the lung.
Moxa heating. Ta-ch'ui (B–1), Fêng-mên (B–4), Fei-yü (B–5). Heating is to be applied only between asthmatic attacks.

Cough

Main points. Fei-yü (B–5), T'ien-t'u (CA–1), Ch'ih-che (UE–20), Lieh-ch'üeh (UE–21), Ch'uan-hsi (B–3).

Rhinitis

Main points. Yin-t'ang (HN–6), Ho-ku (UE–12).
Supplemental points. Yin-hsiang (HN–17).

Pharyngitis, Tonsillitis

Main points. T'ien-yung (HN–30), Ho-ku (UE–12).
Supplemental points. Shao-shang (UE–23), Ch'ü-ch'ih (UE–7).

Hypertension

Main points. Group 1: Ch'ü-ch'ih (UE–7), T'ai-ch'ung (LE–33). Group 2: Fêng-ch'ih (HN–25), Tsu-san-li (LE–10).
Supplemental points. T'ai-yang (HN–3), Yin-t'ang (HN–6), I-fêng (HN–28), Shên-mên (UE–30).

The two main groups may be alternately used. For symptomatic relief, the supplemental points are added: for temporal headache, T'ai-yang; for frontal headache, Yin-t'ang; for tinnitus, I-fêng; and for insomnia, Shên-mên.

Ear points. The point is located at the specific site for the heart.

Nausea and Emesis

Main points. Nei-kuan (UE–26).
Supplemental points. Tsu-san-li (LE–10), Chung-kuan (CA–6).

Gastralgia

Main points. Nei-kuan (UE–26), Tsu-san-li (LE–10).
Supplemental points. Chung-kuan (CA–6), Wei-yü (B–13).
Ear points. The point is located at the specific site for the stomach.
Moxa heating. Chung-kuan (CA–6), Tsu-san-li (LE–10). Heating is performed only between attacks of pain.

Dyspepsia

Main points. Chung-kuan (CA–6), T'ien-shu (CA–12), Ch'i-hai (CA–8), Tsu-san-li (LE–10).
Supplemental points. P'i-yü (B–12), Shêng-yü (B–15), Nei-kuan (UE–26), San-yin-chiao (LE–27).

Ear points. These are located at the specific sites for the stomach, intestines, and gallbladder.
Moxa heating. Any of the above points may be used.

For pediatric digestive disorders, the point Szŭ-fêng (UE–33) is used.

Constipation

Main points. Chih-kou (UE–14), T'ien-shu (CA–12).

Dysentery

Main points. Shang-chü-hsü (LE–12), T'ien-shu (CA–12).
Supplemental points. Nei-kuan (UE–26), Kuan-yüan (CA–9), Ch'ü-ch'ih (UE–7).

Intermittent twirling for 30 minutes is recommended for the point Shang-chü-hsü. The supplemental points Nei-kuan for emesis and Ch'ü-ch'ih for fever are added as necessary. Treatment is performed 1 to 3 times a day.

Ear points. These are located at the sites designated for the small and large intestines.
Moxa heating. Chung-kuan (CA–6), T'ien-shu (CA–12), Ch'i-chung (CA–7), Kuan-yüan (CA–9).

Ileus (paralytic)

Main points. Tsu-san-li (LE–10), Nei-kuan (UE–26).
Ear points. The point is located at the specific site for the intestines.

Hepatitis

Main points. Kan-yü (B–10), Tan-yü (B–11), Tsu-san-li (LE–10), T'ai-ch'ung (LE–33).
Supplemental points. Ta-ch'ui (B–1), I-ming (HN–29), Yang-lin-ch'üan (LE–15).

The supplemental points Ta-ch'ui for fever, I-ming for depression, and Yang-lin-ch'üan for jaundice are added when necessary.

Biliary Colic

Main points. Tan-nang-hsüeh (LE–16), Nei-kuan (UE–26).
Ear points. These are located at the sites designated for the gallbladder and the liver.

Appendicitis

Main points. Lan-wei-hsüeh (LE–11), Ch'ü-ch'ih (UE–7), Nei-t'ing (LE–14).
Supplemental points. T'ien-shu (CA–12).

Intermittent twirling for 1 to 2 hours is recommended. Treatment is performed 2 to 3 times a day until the abdominal pain does not recur.

This treatment is not recommended when appendiceal rupture is suspected.

Enuresis

Main points. Kuan-yüan (CA–9), San-yin-chiao (LE–27).
Supplemental points. Tsu-san-li (LE–10).
Ear points. Located at the specific site for the urinary tract.

Impotence

Main points. Kuan-yüan (CA–9), San-yin-chiao (LE–27).
Supplemental points. Shêng-yü (B–15), Tsu-san-li (LE–10).

Renal Colic

Main points. Shêng-yü (B–15), San-yin-chiao (LE–27).
Supplemental points. Chih-shih (B–16), T'ai-ch'i (LE–34).
Ear points. The point is located at the specific site for the urinary tract.

Urinary Tract Infections

Main points. Ts'ŭ-liao (B–21), San-yin-chiao (LE–27), Chung-chi (CA–10), Ch'ü-ch'üan (LE–31).
Supplemental points. P'ang-k'uang-yü (B–23), Ch'ü-ch'ih (UE–7).
Ear points. The point is located at the site designated for the urinary tract.

Headache

Frontal headache. The acupuncture points are Yin-t'ang (HN–6), Tsuan-tsu (HN–15), Ho-ku (UE–12), T'ai-ch'ung (LE–33).
Temporal headache. The acupuncture points are Fêng-ch'ih (HN–25), T'ai-yang (HN–3), Szŭ-tsu-k'ung (HN–16), Tsu-lin-ch'i (LE–19), Chung-chu (UE–17), Ho-ku (UE–12).
Occipital headache. The acupuncture points are Fêng-ch'ih (HN–25), T'ien-chu (HN–27), Hou-ch'i (UE–18), Shu-ku (LE–23), Ho-ku (UE–12).
Vertical headache. The acupuncture points are Pê-hui (HN–1), Fêng-ch'ih (HN–25), Ho-ku (UE–12), T'ai-ch'ung (LE–33).
Generalized headache. The acupuncture points are Fêng-ch'ih (HN–25), Ho-ku (UE–12), Pê-hui (HN–1), K'un-lun (LE–22).

Toothache

Main points. Ho-ku (UE–12).
Supplemental points. Chia-ch'ê (HN–9), Hsia-kuan (HN–8).

For toothache of the upper teeth, the supplemental point is Hsia-kuan; for the lower teeth, Chia-ch'ê.

Ear points. This point is located at the specific site for the cheek.

Tic Douloureux

Main points. Tsuan-tsu (HN–15), Szŭ-pê (HN–7), Hsia-kuan (HN–8), Chia-ch'êng-chiang (HN–21).
Supplemental points. Ho-ku (UE–12), Nei-t'ing (LE–14), T'ai-ch'ung (LE–33), Tsu-san-li (LE–10).

Opthalmic branch: The point Tsuan-tsu is used.
Maxillary branch: The point Szŭ-pê is used.
Mandibular branch: The points Hsia-kuan and Chia-ch'êng-chiang are used.

Facial Nerve Paralysis

Main points. I-fêng (HN–28), Szŭ-pê (HN–7), Yang-pê (HN–4), Ti-ts'ang (HN–19).
Supplemental points. Jen-chung (HN–18), Chia-ch'êng-chiang (HN–21), T'ai-yang (HN–3), Ho-ku (UE–12).

Poliomyelitis

Main points. Chien-yü (UE–2), Pi-nao (UE–8), Ch'ü-ch'ih (UE–7), and Ho-ku (UE–12) for paralysis of the upper extremities; Huan-t'iao (LE–1), Chih-pien (B–24), Yin-mên (LE–7), Fêng-shih (LE–6), Fu-t'u (LE–5), and Tsu-san-li (LE–10) for paralysis of the lower extremities.
Supplemental points. Chien-liao (UE–4) and Wai-kuan (UE–15) for the upper extremities; Yang-lin-ch'üan (LE–15), Chüeh-ku (LE–17), K'un-lun (LE–22), and T'ai-ch'i (LE–34) for the lower extremities.

For treatment of paralysis, three to six main points and two to four supplemental points are used for each treatment.

Amyotrophia

For the upper extremities. Chien-yü (UE–2), Ch'ü-ch'ih (UE–7), Lieh-ch'üeh (UE–21), T'ai-yüan (UE–22), Ho-ku (UE–12).
For the lower extremities. Tsu-san-li (LE–10), Fêng-shih (LE–6), Huan-t'iao (LE–1), Yang-lin-ch'üan (LE–15), Chiai-ch'i (LE–13), T'ai-yüan (UE–22), Chüeh-ku (LE–17), Fu-t'u (LE–5).

The point Lieh-ch'üeh is specific for weakness of the wrist.

Hemiplegia

Main points. Chien-yü (UE–2), Ch'ü-ch'ih (UE–7), Wai-kuan (UE–15), Ho-ku (UE–12), Huan-t'iao (LE–1), Fêng-shih (LE–6), Yang-lin-ch'üan (LE–15), Chüeh-ku (LE–17), Lien-ch'üan (HN–33).

Two to three of the main points from each afflicted extremity as well as the points Ch'ü-ch'ih and Yang-lin-ch'üan on the normal extremities are utilized in the treatment. The point Lien-ch'üan is specifically indicated for dysarthria.

Epilepsy

Main points. Hsin-yü (B–6), Fei-yü (B–5), P'i-yü (B–12), Ta-ch'ui (B–1).
Supplemental points. Tsu-san-li (LE–10), Nei-kuan (UE–26).

Insomnia

Main points. Shên-mên (UE–30), San-yin-chiao (LE–27).
Supplemental points. Nei-kuan (UE–26), Yin-pê (LE–30), T'ai-ch'i (LE–34).

Neurasthenia

Main points. I-ming (HN–29), Shên-mên (UE–30), San-yin-chiao (LE–27).

Supplemental points. T'ai-yang (HN–3), Pê-hui (HN–1), Nei-kuan (UE–26), Chung-kuan (CA–6), T'ien-shu (CA–12), Kuan-yüan (CA–9), Ts'ŭ-liao (B–21), Tsu-san-li (LE–10).

HYSTERICAL BEHAVIOR

Main points. Jen-chung (HN–18), Nei-kuan (UE–26), Ho-ku (UE–12), T'ai-ch'i (LE–34), San-yin-chiao (LE–27).

This treatment is used in conjunction with orthodox psychiatric therapy.

SCHIZOPHRENIA

Main points. Group 1: Jen-chung (HN–18), Ho-ku (UE–12), T'ai-ch'ung (LE–33). Group 2: T'ai-yang (HN–3), Nei-kuan (UE–26), San-yin-chiao (LE–27).
Supplemental points. Ya-mên (HN–26), Ta-Ch'ui (B–1), T'ao-tao (B–2), T'ing-kung (HN–23), Ching-ming (HN–10).

Treatment is performed once or twice daily using the two groups of main points alternately. Best response is achieved by using all the points in the group simultaneously. Stimulation by twirling is maintained continuously or intermittently for one-half hour. A 26 gauge needle is used. If no response is noted in a week's time, supplemental points are added. As a rule, treatment is continued for a month on a daily basis, even after improvement is noted. Frequency of treatment can then be reduced to a weekly basis.

PELVIC INFLAMMATORY DISEASES,
MENSTRUAL IRREGULARITIES AND CRAMPS

Main points. Kuan-yüan (CA–9), San-yin-chiao (LE–27).
Supplemental points. Ch'i-ch'ung (CA–13), Li-kou (LE–32), Hsüeh-hai (LE–25), Tsu-san-li (LE–10), Yin-lin-ch'üan (LE–26), P'i-yü (B–12), Kung-sun (LE–29).

Ch'i-ch'ung and Li-kou are specific supplemental points for pelvic inflammatory diseases; Hsüeh-hai, Tsu-san-li, and Yin-lin-ch'üan for menstrual irregularities; and Kung-sun for menstrual cramps.

Ear points. Located at the specific sites for the uterus, the ovary, and the hormonal system.

Induction of Labor

Main points. Shang-liao (B–20), Ts'ŭ-liao (B–21), Ho-ku (UE–12), San-yin-chiao (LE–27).

Diseases of the Eye

Main points. Ching-ming (HN–10), Fêng-ch'ih (HN–25), Ho-ku (UE–12).
Supplemental points. T'ai-yang (HN–3), Yang-pê (HN–4), Ch'iu-hou (HN–12), Ch'êng-ch'i (HN–11), Nei-kuan (UE–26), Tsu-san-li (LE–10).

The supplemental point T'ai-yang is added to the main points for the treatment of conjunctivitis and keratitis. Some blood should be produced from this point. For glaucoma, the supplemental points are Yang-pê and T'ai-yang; for optic neuritis and optic nerve atrophy, Ch'iu-hou and Ch'êng-ch'i. *The needle should not be twirled when it is inserted within the orbital rim.* Treatment is performed for 15 to 30 minutes daily for 10 to 15 days; it may then be resumed after a rest period of a week.

Deafness and Mutism

Main points. Êrh-mên (HN–22), T'ing-kung (HN–23), T'ing-hui (HN–24), Ya-mên (HN–26), Lien-ch'üan (HN–33).
Supplemental points. Ho-ku (UE–12), Chung-chu (UE–17), Wai-kuan (UE–15).

For deafness, the main points Êrh-mên, T'ing-kung, and T'ing-hui are used. When response is obtained, the points for mutism, Ya-mên and Lien-ch'üan, are added. In general, two or three of the main points, together with one of the supplemental points, are utilized. Performed once daily, the treatment is continued for 10 days. It is resumed after a rest period of 3 to 7 days. Intensive speech therapy is instituted as soon as the patient can hear.

Tinnitus

Main points. I-fêng (HN–28), I-ming (HN–29), T'ien-yu (HN–31), Fêng-ch'ih (HN–25).
Supplemental points. Chung-chu (UE–17), Wai-kuan (UE–15).

A combination of two main points and one supplemental point is used for each treatment.

Ménière's Disease

Main points. Fêng-ch'ih (HN–25), Nei-kuan (UE–26).
Supplemental points. I-fêng (HN–28), T'ing-kung (HN–23), Tsu-san-li (LE–10), Chung-kuan (CA–6).

The points Tsu-san-li and Chung-kuan are added to the main points when nausea is part of the symptomatology. If hearing is impaired, I-fêng and T'ing-kung should also be used.

Goiter

Main points. Ch'i-yin (HN–34), Ho-ku (UE–12).

Lumbago

Main points. Pressure points.
Supplemental points. Hou-ch'i (UE–18), Yin-mên (LE–7).

Ear points. Located at the specific site for the spinal column.
Moxa heating. Same as acupuncture points.

Best results are obtained by simultaneous application of acupuncture and moxa heating.

Sciatica

Main points. Huan-t'iao (LE–1), Yin-mên (LE–7), Yang-lin-ch'üan (LE–15), pressure points.
Supplemental points. Shang-liao (B–20), Wei-chung (LE–20), Ch'êng-san (LE–21).
Ear points. Located at the specific sites for the spinal column, the kidney, and the point for the sciatic nerve.
Moxa heating. Same points as acupuncture points.

Best results are obtained by simultaneous application of acupuncture and moxa heating.

Painful Disorders, Hip

Main points. Huan-t'iao (LE–1), Chü-liao (LE–2).
Moxa heating. Same as acupuncture points.

Best results are obtained by simultaneous application of acupuncture and moxa heating.

Painful Disorders, Knee

Main points. Nei-wai-ch'i-yen (LE–8), Liang-ch'iu (LE–9), Yang-lin-ch'üan (LE–15), pressure points.
Supplemental points. Wei-chung (LE–20).
Moxa heating. Same as acupuncture points.

Best results are obtained by simultaneous application of acupuncture and moxa heating.

Painful Disorders, Ankle

Main points. Chiai-ch'i (LE–13), Ch'iu-hsü (LE–18), pressure points.
Supplemental points. Chüeh-ku (LE–17).
Moxa heating. Same as acupuncture points.

Best results are obtained by simultaneous application of acupuncture and moxa heating.

Painful Disorders, Toe

Main points. Pa-fêng (LE–37), Shang-pa-fêng (LE–38).
Moxa heating. Same as acupuncture points.

Best results are obtained by simultaneous application of acupuncture and moxa heating.

Painful Disorders, Heel and Sole of Foot

Main points. Pressure points.
Supplemental points. Ch'êng-san (LE–21), T'ai-ch'i (LE–34).
Moxa heating. Same as acupuncture points.

Best results are obtained by simultaneous application of acupuncture and moxa heating.

Painful Disorders, Shoulder

Main points. Chien-yü (UE–2), Chien-liao (UE–4), Nao-yü (UE–5), T'ien-tsung (B–9), Chien-nei-lin (UE–3), Chü-ku (UE–1), pressure points.
Supplemental points. Ch'ü-yüan (B–8), Pi-nao (UE–8), Yang-lin-ch'üan (LE–15).

For subscapular bursitis, the main points to be used are T'ien-tsung, Nao-yü, and Chien-nei-lin.

For subacromial bursitis, the main points recommended are Chien-yü, and Chien-liao.

For supraspinatus tendinitis, the main points are Chien-yü, and Chü-ku.

For tendinitis of the long head of the biceps muscle, pressure points are the main points.

In all of the above conditions, addition of the supplemental point, Yang-lin-ch'üan, is desirable.

Treatment is carried out every other day for a total of 7 to 10 treatments. If necessary, treatment may be resumed after a rest period of a week. Best results are obtained by simultaneous application of acupuncture and moxa heating.

Ear points. They are located at the specific site for the shoulder.
Moxa heating. Same as the acupuncture points.

Painful Disorders, Elbow

Main points. Ch'ü-ch'ih (UE–7), T'ien-ching (UE–13), Chou-liao (UE–10), pressure points.
Supplemental points. Yang-lin-ch'üan (LE–15).
Moxa heating. Same as the acupuncture points.

Best results are obtained by simultaneous application of acupuncture and moxa heating.

Painful Disorders, Wrist

Main points. Yang-ch'ih (UE–16), Wai-kuan (UE–15), pressure points.
Supplemental points. Yang-ch'i (UE–11), T'ai-yüan (UE–22), Lieh-ch'üeh (UE–21).

For deQuervain's disease (stenosing tenosynovitis over the radial styloid), the main points are the pressure points. The supplemental points are Yang-ch'i, T'ai-yüan, and Lieh-ch'üeh.

For median nerve compression at the wrist, the main points are Ta-lin (UE–27), Shang-pa-hsieh (UE–32), and Nei-kuan (UE–26).

Moxa heating. Same as the acupuncture points.

PAINFUL DISORDERS, FINGER JOINTS

Main points. Pa-hsieh (UE–31), Shang-pa-hsieh (UE–32).

PAINFUL DISORDERS, MANDIBULAR JOINTS

Main points. Hsia-kuan (HN–8), Ho-ku (UE–12).

TORTICOLLIS

Main points. Pressure points in the neck and shoulders.
Supplemental points. Fêng-ch'ih (HN–25), Chüeh-ku (LE–17), Hou-ch'i (UE–18).

ISCHEMIA OF THE EXTREMITIES

Main points. Ch'ü-ch'ih (UE–7) and Shao-hai (UE–29) for upper extremities; Yang-lin-ch'üan (LE–15) and Yin-lin-ch'üan (LE–26) for the lower extremities.
Supplemental points. Shang-pa-hsieh (UE–32) for the upper extremities; Shang-pa-fêng (LE–38) for the lower extremities.
Moxa heating. Same as the acupuncture points.

This treatment is indicated for conditions such as intermittent claudication and Raynaud's disease.

NEURODERMATITIS

Main points. Ch'ü-ch'ih (UE–7), Hsüeh-hai (LE–25).
Supplemental points. Ho-ku (UE–12), San-yin-chiao (LE–27).
Ear points. Located at the specific sites for the lung, the liver, and the adrenal glands.
Moxa heating. Same as the acupuncture points.

ACUPUNCTURE-ANESTHESIA

5 ACUPUNCTURE-ANESTHESIA

Among the many contributions of contemporary medicine in the People's Republic of China, perhaps the most impressive achievement is the development of acupuncture-anesthesia, an accomplishment that truly reflects the successful integration of traditional Chinese medicine with Western science. Since its discovery in 1958, acupuncture-anesthesia has been safely utilized in more than 700,000 surgical operations with a success rate of approximately 90 percent. It varies in effectiveness mainly in the type of operation performed. Its advantages over conventional anesthesia in terms of tolerance, safety, economics, and simplicity are obvious. A patient "under" acupuncture-anesthesia is free of pain, but his other physiological functions remain unimpaired. He is conscious and mentally alert, allowing, in certain operations, the advantage of cooperation between surgeon and patient. Obviated are the postoperative complications and discomforts that attend conventional anesthesia.

Extensive clinical research in acupuncture-anesthesia has been conducted, and is continuing, in China and in some European countries, notably Soviet Russia. Suffice it to say that there is no scientific theory to date that can entirely explain all the physiological effects of acupuncture-anesthesia. There is, however, general agreement that different levels of the central nervous system are involved and that other systems, such as the humoral system, may also be participating factors.

PRINCIPLES OF ACUPUNCTURE-ANESTHESIA

The technique of needle insertion for acupuncture-anesthesia is similar to the technique described for the treatment of disease. There are certain salient features, however, that are considered highly essential for the induction of acupuncture-anesthesia. First, it is imperative to obtain a strong sensory response (Te-ch'i) to acupuncture. This response must be maintained throughout the period of induction and anesthesia by continuous stimulation of the acupuncture points. Second, an induction or stimulation period of at least 20 to 30 minutes is advised in order to attain surgical anesthesia. Although continuous stimulation of the points may be performed by manual twirling combined with a rapid up-and-down movement of the needles, it is more practical to stimulate the points mechanically by attaching the needles to electrodes connected to a phasic battery power unit. The latter serves strictly as a labor-saving device and is especially advantageous in situations where multiple needles are inserted, in long surgical procedures, and in situations where operating space is limited and the acupuncture needles are, of necessity, inserted in the vicinity of the operative field.

Premedication may or may not be given, nor is it found essential for anesthesia. The patients are reassured and informed of what to expect. To compensate for possible respiratory embarrassment in chest operations such as thoracotomy and pulmonary resection, patients undergoing these operations are taught to "breathe with their abdominal muscles" for several days prior to surgery.

Throughout surgery, the patient's vital signs—pulse, respiration, blood pressure—should be closely monitored. During the operation, an analgesic, hypnotic, sedative, or local anesthetic may be added to supplement acupuncture-anesthesia when indicated. Standard anesthesia equipment should also be available nearby in the event that conventional anesthesia is required for completion of the surgery.

In operations utilizing acupuncture-anesthesia, deftness in surgical technique is mandatory. The incisions should be executed with light, quick, and precise strokes and every effort should be made to handle the tissues gently.

The analgesic effect of acupuncture-anesthesia does not end with cessation of the stimulation for the anesthesia but persists for several hours thereafter. When it finally recedes, it may again be induced by acupuncture. Except for occasional ecchymoses at the acupuncture sites, no post-anesthetic side effects or untoward reactions directly attributable to acupuncture-anesthesia have been reported.

SELECTION OF ACUPUNCTURE POINTS

Body points. Most acupuncture points for anesthesia are selected from the traditional acupuncture points described in Chapters 2 and 3. As a rule, this selection is based on knowing precisely which area or organ of the human anatomy is directly affected by stimulation of a specific acupuncture point. Thus, since pharyngitis, tonsillitis, and toothaches are relieved by stimulation of the point Ho-ku, it followed that this point would be used to induce anesthesia for surgery in the region of the pharynx and the mouth. Indeed, this was the point utilized for the first tonsillectomy performed under acupuncture-anesthesia. Similarly, Kung-sun and San-yin-chiao, two of several acupuncture points employed for the relief of abdominal disorders, are logically among those selected for acupuncture-anesthesia for abdominal operations. In a like manner, points for appendectomy (Lan-wei-hsüeh and T'ien-shu) and for thyroidectomy (San-yang-lo and Fuh-t'u) were identified. The former point, used in conjunction with the point I-fêng, also provides excellent anesthesia for chest operations such as thoracotomy and pneumonectomy.

Ear points. These points are very frequently utilized for acupuncture-anesthesia, either by themselves or in combination with acupuncture points in other locations. As in the treatment of diseases where each diseased organ or body area is treated by stimulating the acupuncture point located at its specific site at the external ear, anesthesia for the organ or area in question would be induced by the use of the appropriate ear point. Examples of combinations of ear points employed to achieve anesthesia for various surgical procedures are given in Table 23. These points are identified in Fig. 48. Several recent clinical studies to evaluate the efficacy of injecting various substances into the ear points to provide surgical anesthesia have reportedly yielded promising results. Included were injections of small quantities (0.1 to 0.2 cc.) of extracts of Chinese herbs and Vitamin B_1 into the organ-specific points in both ears.

Table 23

COMBINATIONS OF ACUPUNCTURE POINTS FOR ACUPUNCTURE–ANESTHESIA IN VARIOUS OPERATIONS

OPERATION OR SITE OF OPERATION	ACUPUNCTURE POINTS
Brain or cranial operations	1. Chüan-liao 2. Chüan-liao, Tsu-lin-chi, T'ai-ch'ung, Hsien-ku 3. Ear Points: Shên-mên to Kidney, Brain to Subcortex, Chiao-kan, Lung 4. Ho-ku, Nei-kuan Ear Points: Shên-mên to Kidney, Neck
Ophthalmic surgery	1. Ho-ku, Nei-kuan 2. Ho-ku, Tsuan-tsu to Yü-yao, Szŭ-pê 3. Ho-ku, Tsuan-tsu Ear Points: Shên-mên, Lung 4. Ho-ku Ear Points: Eye-1 to Eye-2, Lung 5. Ho-ku, Chih-kou Ear Points: Shên-mên, Chiao-kan, Eye-1, Eye-2
Ear, nose, and oral surgery including dental procedures	1. Ho-ku 2. Ho-ku, Nei-kuan, Nei-ting 3. Ho-ku, Yin-hsiang 4. Ho-ku, Hou-ch'i 5. Ear Points: Anesthetic points for tooth extraction

OPERATION OR SITE OF OPERATION	ACUPUNCTURE POINTS	
Neck operations including tonsillectomy, thyroidectomy, laryngectomy, radical neck dissection	1. Fuh-t'u (thyroidectomy) 2. Ho-ku, Nei-kuan 3. Ho-ku, Nei-kuan Ear Points: Shên-mên, Chiao-kan, Lung, Neck 4. Ho-ku, Chih-kou Ear Points: Shên-mên to Chiao-kan, Lung, Adrenal gland to Pharynx, Neck to P'ing-ch'uan	
Thoracic surgery including pulmonary, cardiac, and mediastinal operations	1. Ho-ku, Nei-kuan 2. San-yang-lo, I-fêng 3. Ear Points: Shên-mên, Lung, Chest, Heart, Chiao-kan 4. Pi-nao	
Abdominal operations including gastric surgery, cholecystectomy splenectomy, intestinal operations, appendectomy, and herniorraphy	1. Tsu-san-li, Shang-chü-hsü, Nei-kuan 2. Ear Points: Stomach, Shên-mên Chiao-kan, Lung	Gastric surgery
	3. Tsu-san-li, San-yin-chiao, Tan-nang-hsüeh 4. Ho-ku, Nei-kuan Ear Points: Shên-mên to Gall-bladder, Chiao-kan, Lung Abdomen	Cholecystectomy
	5. Tsu-san-li, San-yin-chiao, T'ai-ch'ung 6. Ear Points: Chiao-kan, Shên-mên, Lung,	Splenectomy

OPERATION OR SITE OF OPERATION	ACUPUNCTURE POINTS	
Abdominal operations including gastric surgery, cholecystectomy splenectomy, intestinal operations, appendectomy, and herniorraphy	Spleen, Abdomen Nose Points: Lung, Ear, Spleen	Splenectomy
	7. Tsu-san-li, Kung-sun or T'ai-ch'ung, Ho-ku, Nei-kuan	Intestinal surgery
	8. Tsu-san-li 9. Lan-wei-hsüeh 10. Ear Points: Appendix, Lung, Shên-mên, Abdomen	Appendectomy
Gynecological surgery including hysterectomy, Caesarean-section, tubal ligation	1. Tsu-san-li, Tai-mo 2. Tsu-san-li, Tai-mo, San-yin-chiao 3. Ear Points: Uterus, Shên-mên, Abdomen, Lung, Chiao-kan	
Genitourinary operations including renal, ureteral, urinary bladder, scrotal or testicular surgery, and cystoscopy	1. Tsu-san-li, San-yin-chiao 2. San-yin-chiao, Li-kou 3. Ear Points: Lung, Shên-mên, Chiao-kan, Abdomen, Kidney or Bladder	
Shoulder surgery	1. Wai-kuan, Hsi-mên, Kung-tsui, Ho-ku 2. Ear Points: Shoulder to Shoulder joint, Shên-mên, Chiao-kan, Kidney 3. Ho-ku, Kung-tsui Ear Points: Shoulder to Shoulder joint, Lung, Kidney, Shên-mên to Chiao-kan	
Upper arm operations	1. Ch'u-ch'ih, Ho-ku 2. Ho-ku, Chung-chu Ear Points: Elbow, Shên-mên	
Elbow surgery	1. Chien-yü, Chien-nei-lin, Ho-ku, Wai-kuan, Ch'u-ch'ih Ear Points: Elbow to Shoulder, Shên-mên, Kidney, Spleen to Lung	

OPERATION OR SITE OF OPERATION	ACUPUNCTURE POINTS
Forearm operations	1. Ho-ku, Ch'u-ch'ih, Chien-yü, Nao-yü Ear Points: Elbow to Wrist, Lung, Shên-mên 2. Nei-kuan Ear Points: Elbow to Wrist, Lung, Kidney
Hip operations	1. Nei-t'ing, Shêng-yü, T'ai-ch'i 2. Yang-lin-ch'üan, Tsu-san-li Ear Points: Lung to Subcortex, Shên-mên to Chiao-kan, Kidney
Thigh surgery	1. Tsu-san-li, K'un-lun 2. Tsu-san-li, Fêng-lung, Chüeh-ku, San-yin-chiao, Ch'iu-hsu, Hsien-ku 3. Yang-lin-ch'üan, Chüeh-ku, Chung-tu, Fêng-lung 4. Ear Points: Hip to Ankle, Shên-mên, Lung, Chiao-kan, Kidney, Adrenal gland
Knee surgery	1. Fêng-shih, Yang-lin-ch'üan, Yin-lin-ch'üan, Yin-mên, Ta-ch'ang-yü, Ch'i-hai-yü
Leg operations	1. Huan-t'iao, Chih-pien Ear Points: Knee to Ankle, Shên-mên, Lung 2. T'ai-ch'ung, Yin-lin-ch'üan, Hsüeh-hai, Huan-t'iao Ear Points: Knee to Ankle, Subcortex
Lumbar operations	1. Ho-ku, Wai-kuan, Points 1.5 inches lateral to the beginning and the end of the incision Ear Points: Shên-mên to Chiao-kan, Vertebrae, Lung, Kidney 2. Ear Points: Vertebrae, Subcortex, Chiao-kan, Shên-mên to Kidney

NOTES: For needling of multiple points or "point to point" (e.g., Elbow to Shoulder, Spleen to Lung), see technique of needle insertion described in the section on Nose Points, below.

Needles inserted at points in the operative field may be removed after anesthesia has been induced and stimulation of the remaining points continued all through surgery.

All points listed are Body Points unless otherwise indicated.

See Fig. 48 for locations of Ear Points.

Nose points. Acupuncture points for every organ or area of the body are also found on the nose (Fig. 52). These points are mainly used for acupuncture-anesthesia. The following report from the People's Hospital, Tseng-chen County, Canton Province (1972), describes the effectiveness of selected nose points in providing acupuncture-anesthesia for various surgical operations (Table 24). The selected nose points utilized in this report were:

1. The lung point, located at the midpoint between the eyebrows.
2. The heart point, located at the midpoint between the medial canthus of the eyes.
3. The liver point, located 0.5 cm. directly below the heart point.
4. The supplemental point #1, located at the upper end of the alar fold of the nose.
5. The supplemental point #2, located between the tip and the alar of the nose.
6. The point Ts'ang-hsin-hsüeh, located midway between the nostrils, at the level of their upper margins and directly below the point for the reproductive organs.
7. The point Tsŭ-pao-hsüeh, located at the anterior nasal spine.

Acupuncture of these selected nose points was accomplished in the following manner: Only four needles were employed for all the points. The first needle was horizontally inserted in a cephalo-caudad direction, beginning slightly above the lung point, passing through the heart point, and terminating at the liver point, embracing all three of these points. The insertion was facilitated by depressing the nose. Also with the nose depressed, the second needle was horizontally inserted, passing from supplemental point #1 to supplemental point #2. In similar manner, a third needle was inserted for the contralateral supplemental points. For the insertion of the fourth needle, the tip of the nose was tilted upwards. The needle was then passed through the columella, beginning at the point Ts'ang-hsin-hsüeh and incorporating and ending at the point Tsŭ-pao-hsüeh.

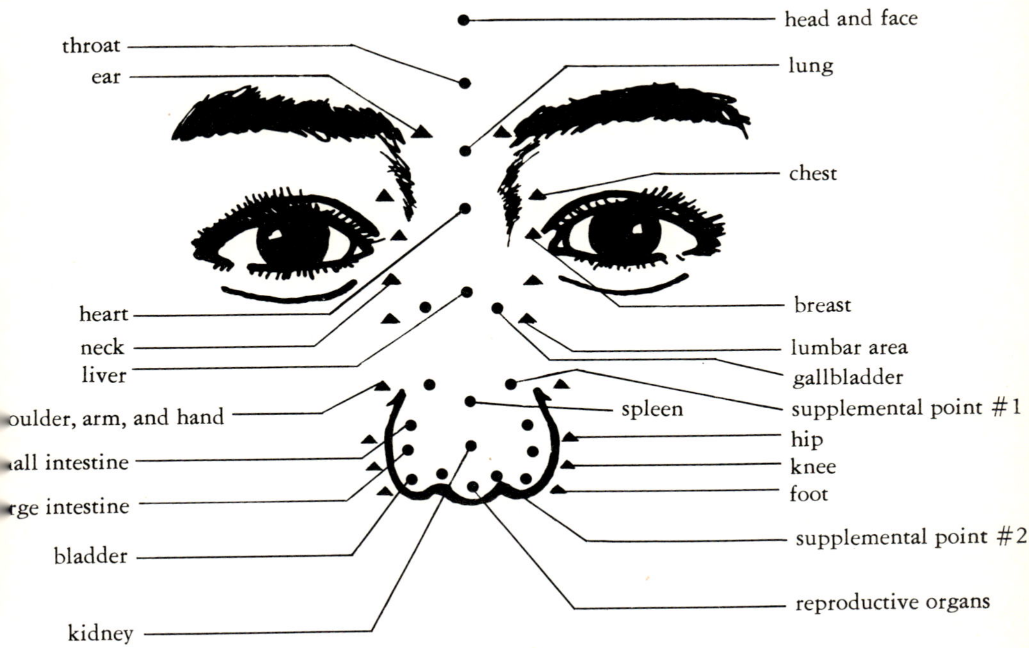

Fig. 52
Acupuncture points of the nose

Table 24

EFFICACY OF ACUPUNCTURE-ANESTHESIA WITH NOSE POINTS

OPERATION	TOTAL No. of cases	TOTAL % success	EXCELLENT No. of cases	EXCELLENT %	GOOD No. of cases	FAIR No. of cases	FAILURE No. of cases
Gastrectomy, gastroenterostomy, intestinal operations	180	99.4	131	72.7	25	23	1
Splenectomy	13	92.3	8	61.5	2	2	1
Cholecystectomy, common duct exploration	7	100.00			7		
Nephrectomy, ureterolithotomy, cystolithotomy, prostatectomy, cystorraphy, cystectomy	16	100.0	8	50.0	7	2	
Hysterectomy, Caesarean section, tubal ligation, oophorectomy	60	98.3	42	70.7	11	6	1
Appendectomy, exploratory laparotomy	26	100.0	9	34.6	13	4	
Thyroidectomy	21	100.0	13	61.9	7	1	

I. Excellent = Acupuncture-anesthesia alone was sufficient.
II. Good = Hypnotics, sedatives, or analgesics were added to supplement acupuncture-anesthesia.
III. Fair = Local anesthetic was added to I and II.
IV. Failure = Conventional anesthesia was needed for completion of operation.
V. % success = Includes excellent, good, and fair results

Selection of Points

In general, acupuncture-anesthesia for a particular surgical procedure is achieved by stimulation of not just only a single acupuncture point but a combination of several points. However, it has been observed in retrospect that during the early stages of the development of acupuncture-anesthesia, frequently more than the necessary number of points was employed to induce anesthesia for a specific operation. Through clinical experience, the trend has been to reduce the necessary number of points whenever feasible. Directly related to this effort is the recent observation that the stimulation of just one point, San-yang-lo, is sufficient to induce anesthesia for thyroidectomy and chest operations.

There is, reportedly, no absolute contraindication to the use of acupuncture-anesthesia. However, apprehensive patients are considered poor candidates for this type of anesthesia. Inadequate muscle relaxation and patient discomfort with traction on the viscera have been significant drawbacks in abdominal operations when acupuncture-anesthesia was used. In these operations, acupuncture-anesthesia is not recommended for patients who have thick abdominal musculature and when considerable visceral traction is anticipated, as could occur in the presence of extensive adhesions. Incomplete analgesia of the skin, the pleura, and the peritoneum occurs in a small percentage of patients, but it is easily remedied by infiltrating the site of the incision with a local anesthetic.

This form of anesthesia is considered most effective for surgical procedures of the head, neck, and chest. It is employed in infants as well as the aged and is ideally suited for patients of high surgical risk, due either to debilitation or serious concurrent diseases. It has also been successfully used in operations on patients who were in shock. In these situations, it was observed that acupuncture helped to raise the blood pressure (10 to 30 mm. Hg in most cases, 50 to 70 in a few) reduced the amount of blood transfused, and also exerted a salutory effect on the functions of the body. Observations relating to the use of acupuncture-anesthesia in various surgical procedures follow.

Neurosurgery. An analysis of the results of 1,101 neurosurgical operations performed under acupuncture-anesthesia at the Peking Hsuan Wu Hospital and the Shanghai First Medical College revealed that the effectiveness of the anesthesia varied with the site of the incision and the type of operation performed—it being most effective in frontal procedures, less so in occipitoparietal operations, and least effective in surgery of the spinal cord. The efficacy of this type of anesthesia was more marked when acupuncture points located in close proximity to the operative site were used, rather than those situated at a distant location (e.g., points of the extremities). Some problems encountered include incomplete analgesia of the skin in some cases requiring the use of local anesthetics, reactions of nausea, emesis, and diaphoresis secondary to traction on the dura mater and the diaphragma sellae necessitating the use of drugs or acupuncture of the points Nei-kuan and T'ai-ch'ung for relief, and the occasional occurrence of the syndrome of low intracranial pressure. The latter may be remedied by lowering the head of the patient and by stimulating the points San-yin-chiao and Fu-liu. On the positive side, the results showed that with acupuncture-anesthesia there was minimal interference with the physiological functions of the patient, immediate assessment of the operative result was feasible, and postoperative nursing care easier.

Thyroidectomy. The use of acupuncture-anesthesia in thyroidectomy has been highly successful, with the rate of success exceeding 90% in most series. At the Shanghai First People's Hospital, where over 700 cases of thyroidectomies have been performed under anesthesia induced by acupuncture, excellent anesthesia was obtained in 95% of the operations when the point Fuh-t'u was used. However, despite these impressive statistics, incomplete analgesia of the skin occurs in a few cases and pain from ligation of the thyroid arteries and from traction on the gland, remains a problem. Respiratory difficulty from tracheal compression or obstruction may also be encountered. Precautionary measures suggested for avoiding this serious difficulty include administration of drugs to reduce tracheal secretions, proper positioning of the patient for surgery, and early separation of muscles that may be compressing an enlarged thyroid gland against the trachea.

Laryngectomy. Using ear and body points, surgical anesthesia was successfully induced in 91.9% of 74 cases of laryngectomies performed at the Shanghai First Medical College. The advantages of performing laryngectomy with acupuncture-anesthesia included minimal systemic reactions, less tracheal secretions during and after the operation, easy evaluation of the suturing of the pharyngolaryngeal mucous membrane, and a more speedy recovery. As with thyroidectomy, pain from traction on the larynx, an annoying cough, incompleteness of analgesia, and difficult breathing occasionally occurred.

Thoracic operations. Acupuncture-anesthesia was entirely satisfactory in close to 90% of hundreds of intrathoracic operations carried out in hospitals in Peking and Shanghai. The surgical procedures included pulmonary resections, decortication, patent ductus operations, cardiac surgery such as valvulotomy of the mitral valve, resections of mediastinal tumors, and radical operations for cancer of the esophagus and the cardia of the stomach. Acupuncture points selected for anesthesia for these procedures include those enumerated in Table 23.

As earlier mentioned, patients undergoing thoracic operations were instructed preoperatively on deep abdominal breathing, a maneuver for controlling or alleviating mediastinal flutter and paradoxical respiration that may occur following opening of the chest. During surgery, troublesome cough reflexes were suppressed by deep open-mouth inspiration or by peribronchial infiltration of a local anesthetic. In some instances, endotracheal intubation was necessary to clear the respiratory tract of excessive bronchial secretions or to assist respiration. Acupuncture-anesthesia was employed not only in patients with normal pulmonary function but also for those with impaired function.

Splenectomy. A review of 305 cases of splenectomies carried out under anesthesia induced by acupuncture at the Ch'angshan County People's Hospital, Chekiang, China, revealed that good to excellent anesthesia was achieved in 95.5% of the operations. Ear and nose points were employed (see Table 23). The results indicate that stimulation of the ear points strongly suppressed the unpleasant sensations of traction on the organs while comparatively more satisfactory muscular relaxation and analgesia were obtained from needling of the nose points. Additional muscular relaxation was provided by infiltrating 10 to 30 cc. of a local anesthetic into the muscles during the operation. When necessary, an intravenous drip of an analgesic (e.g., Demerol) was also administered for incomplete analgesia.

Pediatric surgery. At the Peking Children's Hospital, 1,308 children, ranging in age from 1 day to 14 years, have undergone various surgical procedures under acupuncture-anesthesia. Highly satisfactory anesthesia was obtained in approximately 80% of the operations. Prior to receiving acupuncture, most of the children were given some form of sedation. In that children do find the sensory response to acupuncture (Te-ch'i) quite disagreeable, ear points are more frequently utilized than body points for acupuncture-anesthesia in pediatric surgery, and effectively so. Unpleasant reactions from traction on the muscles and inadequate muscle relaxation are lesser problems with pediatric patients probably because of reduced muscle mass.

Although much experimentation is still in progress in the field of acupuncture-anesthesia, this type of anesthesia is at present considered the anesthetic of choice in China when conditions favor its use. It is, nevertheless, regarded only as an addition to, and not as a replacement for, other forms of anesthesia.

CURRENT CHINESE OBSERVATIONS ON THE MECHANISM(S) OF ACUPUNCTURE-ANALGESIA

In the last few years, intensive research studies on acupuncture-analgesia have been carried out, and are continuing, in several medical colleges and research institutes in China. These experiments, performed both on humans and laboratory animals, were conducted by neurophysiologists, biologists, and physicians, employing basic scientific methods and parameters. From these endeavors, the following observations and hypotheses have been made.

The analgesic effect of acupuncture is mediated via neural pathways involving at least the peripheral nerves, pain receptors in the substantia gelatinosa of the posterior horn of the spinal cord, in the reticular formation of the midbrain, and in the parafascicularis and the centralis lateralis nuclei of the thalamus. Studies in which microelectrodes were inserted into these pain centers to measure their electrical response to painful stimuli clearly demonstrated that acupuncture will exert a marked inhibitory effect on the response of these receptors to pain.

Further suggestions that acupuncture stimuli are neurologically transmitted are furnished by observations from the following clinical experiments. In hemiplegic patients, it was observed that stimulation of acupuncture points in their normal extremities would significantly elevate their pain threshold, whereas needling of acupuncture points in the affected or paralytic limbs failed to do so. In other experiments involving "neural blockage," stimulation of acupuncture points that had been infiltrated with a local anesthetic produced little or no effect on the ability of the subjects to tolerate pain. Likewise, it was possible to inhibit the analgesic effect of acupuncture by blocking afferent acupuncture impulses with epidural anesthesia. Stemming from the results of these experiments is also the implication that the functional state of the nervous system may well affect the efficacy of acupuncture-analgesia.

Convincing experimental evidence has been produced to indicate that the effect of acupuncture-analgesia is mediated via deep sensory fibers (i.e., through proprioceptors and proprioceptive pathways) rather than by cutaneous ones. For instance, it was noted that while anesthetization of the skin produced minimal or no effect, infiltration of local anesthetics into the "deep nerve supply to the muscles at the acupuncture site" inhibited the analgesic effect of acupuncture. It was further observed that even though several forms of stimuli, including those of pressure, vibration, touch and pinch, could elevate pain threshold to some degree, only the deep sensory afferent impulses of acupuncture, "presumably involving proprioceptors and proprioceptive pathways," significantly reduced pain perception.

Although the exact neurological mechanism of acupuncture-analgesia remains to be solved, the Chinese researchers have offered an attractive hypothesis which postulates that the analgesic effect of acupuncture is the result of an interaction between two different sets of afferent impulses, one set of which arises from the site of pain and the other from the stimulated acupuncture point. Through this interaction, which is believed to be a form of competitive inhibition, pain impulses are blocked out and perception of the intensity and quality of pain subsequently reduced or eliminated.

In the search for a logical or acceptable explanation of acupuncture-analgesia, neurohumoral and neurochemical theories have also been examined. Experiments were devised to determine whether acupuncture would trigger the release of humoral factors or chemicals which, in turn, may affect pain perception. In one such experiment, the circulation of the upper extremity of a group of human subjects was occluded with an inflated sphygmomanometer cuff and acupuncture points distal to the site of occlusion stimulated. A significant elevation of the pain threshold of the subject was noted, a finding that by definition would negate the role of hormones. However, another study performed on rabbits has yielded results to the contrary. In this experiment, cross-circulation by vascular anastomosis was established in pairs of rabbits. Acupuncture, performed on one of each pair of the animals, was found to increase the pain threshold of both rabbits, strongly suggesting that neurohumoral mechanism is indeed involved in acupuncture-analgesia.

Finally, from Peking Medical College comes the report of a possibly significant experiment. Artificial cerebrospinal fluid, first perfused through the ventricle of a rabbit receiving acupuncture, and then infused into the ventricle of a non-accupunctured rabbit, produced a marked rise in the pain threshold of the recipient rabbit. This finding lends some credence to the hypothesis that certain chemicals with the potential of inhibiting pain may well be released in the brain during acupuncture. By adding and subtracting various chemicals to the perfusate, the investigators were also able to study the role and effect of each of these chemicals in acupuncture-analgesia (see Fig. 53).

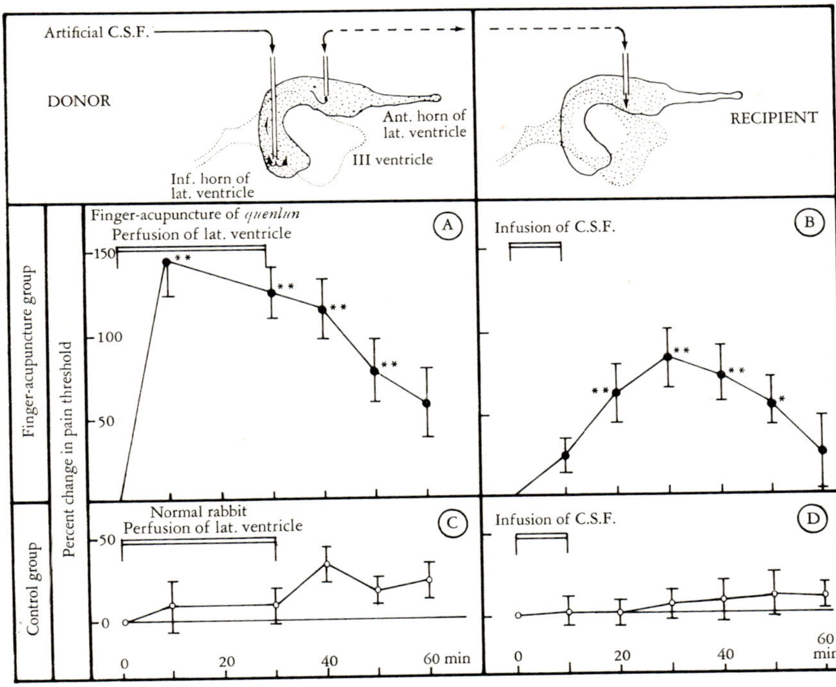

Fig. 53
The effect of finger-acupuncture analgesia in cerebrospinal fluid perfusion experiments

BIBLIOGRAPHY

BIBLIOGRAPHY

SOURCES

With the exception of the Preface and the Introduction, the information in this text was compiled and translated from the publications listed below.

Acupuncture Anesthesia Co-ordinating Group of Shanghai College of Traditional Chinese Medicine, et al. "The Role of Midbrain Reticular Formation in Acupuncture Anesthesia." *Chinese Medical Journal,* no. 3 (1973): 136–38.

Acupuncture Anesthesia Research Group, Hunan Medical College, Changsha. "The Relation between Acupuncture Analgesia and Neurotransmitters in Rabbit Brain." *Chinese Medical Journal,* no. 8 (1973): 478–86.

Chang, H. T. "Integrative Action of Thalamus in the Process of Acupuncture for Analgesia." *Scientia Sinica* 16 (no. 1, 1973): 25–60.

Ch'angshan County People's Hospital, Ch'angshan, Chekiang. "Acupuncture Anesthesia in Splenectomy—Report of 305 Cases." *Chinese Medical Journal,* no. 2 (1973): 90.

Chên Chiu Chih Liao Hsüeh [*Treatment by Acupuncture and Moxibustion*]. Edited by School of Chinese Traditional Medicine, Shanghai, 1960.

針灸治療學 - 上海市中医學院編

Chên Chiu Chih Liao Shou Ts'e [*Handbook of Acupuncture and Moxibustion Treatment*]. Edited by Academy of Acupuncture, Shanghai, 1971.

針灸治療手册 - 上海市針灸研究所編

Chên Chiu Hsüeh [*Acupuncture and Moxibustion*], Edited by School of Chinese Traditional Medicine, Shanghai, May, 1974.
针灸学 - 上海中医学院 编

Chên Chiu Lin Ch'uang Ch'ü Hsüeh T'u Chiai [*Diagrammatic Illustrations of Acupuncture and Moxibustion Points*]. Edited by School of Chinese Traditional Medicine, Peking, 1971.
针灸臨床取穴圖解 - 北京中医學院編

Chên Chiu Yü Hsüeh Hsüeh [*Locations of Acupuncture and Moxibustion Points*]. Edited by School of Chinese Traditional Medicine, Shanghai, 1960.
针灸腧穴學 - 上海市中医學院編

Chiang, C. Y., C. T. Chang, H. L. Chu, and L. F. Yang: "Peripheral Afferent Pathway for Acupuncture Analgesia." *Scientia Sinica* 16 (no. 2, 1973): 210–17.

Chung I Tsa Chih [*Journal of Chinese Medicine*], no. 10, 1959.
中医杂志

Department of Anesthesiology, Hsuan Wu Hospital, Peking. "Acupuncture Anesthesia in Neurosurgery." *Chinese Medical Journal,* no. 2 (1973): 67–70.

Department of Anesthesiology, Teaching Hospital of Anhwei Medical College, Hofei, Anhwei. "Acupuncture Anesthesia for Operations in Shock and Critical Cases." *Chinese Medical Journal,* no. 2 (1973): 95–97.

Department of Physiology, Shanghai First Medical College, et al. "Acupuncture Sensation and Electromyogram of the Needled Point in Patients with Nervous Diseases." *Chinese Medical Journal,* no. 10 (1973): 619–22.

Department of Surgery, Peking Children's Hospital. "Acupuncture Anesthesia in Pediatric Surgery—Report of 1,308 Cases." *Chinese Medical Journal,* no. 2 (1973): 91–94.

Eye, Ear, Nose and Throat Hospital of Shanghai First Medical College. "Laryngectomy under Acupuncture Anesthesia." *Chinese Medical Journal,* no. 2 (1973): 78–79.

Sources

Hsin I Hsüeh [*New Medicine*], no. 9, 1971. 新医學

Hsin I Hsüeh [*New Medicine*], no. 10, 1971.

Hsin I Hsüeh [*New Medicine*], no. 4, 1972.

Hua Shan Hospital of Shanghai First Medical College. "Observations on Analgesic Effect of Needling Chuan-liao point in Neurosurgery—Report of 619 Cases." *Chinese Medical Journal,* no. 2 (1973): 71–73.

Morphologic Section of the Acupuncture Anesthesia Research Unit, Shenyang Medical College. "Preliminary Experimental Morphologic and Electron Microscopic Studies of the Connection between Acupuncture Points on the Limbs and the Segments of the Spinal Cord." *Chinese Medical Journal,* no. 3 (1973): 144–50.

Peking Acupuncture Anesthesia Co-ordinating Group, "Preliminary Study on the Mechanism of Acupuncture Anesthesia." *Scientia Sinica* 16 (no. 3, 1973): 447–56.

Peking Review, Feb. 1972.

Research Group of Acupuncture Anesthesia, Peking Medical College. "Effect of Acupuncture on Pain Threshold of Human Skin." *Chinese Medical Journal,* no. 3 (1973): 151–57.

Research Group of Acupuncture Anesthesia, Peking Medical College. "The Role of Some Neurotransmitters of Brain in Finger-Acupuncture Analgesia." *Scientia Sinica* 17 no. 1 (1974): 112–30.

Section of Thoracic Surgery, Peking Acupuncture Anesthesia Co-ordinating Group. "Acupuncture Anesthesia in Thoracic Surgery—Clinical Analysis of 818 Cases." *Chinese Medical Journal,* no. 2 (1973): 85–88.

Shanghai Acupuncture Research Group, eds. *Acupuncture Anesthesia.* Shanghai Jen-min Ch'u-pan She, 1972.

Shanghai First People's Hospital. "Acupuncture Anesthesia in Thyroidectomy." *Chinese Medical Journal,* no. 2 (1973): 74–77.

Shanghai First Tuberculosis Hospital. "Pulmonary Resections under Acupuncture Anesthesia." *Chinese Medical Journal,* no. 2 (1973): 80–84.

Shanghai Institute of Physiology. "Electrical Response to Nocuous Stimulation and Its Inhibition in Nucleus Centralis Lateralis of Thalamus in Rabbits." *Chinese Medical Journal,* no. 3 (1973): 131–35.

Thoracic Section, Acupuncture Anesthesia Group, Second Teaching Hospital of Hunan Medical College, Changsha, Hunan. "Acupuncture Anesthesia in Cardiac Surgery." *Chinese Medical Journal,* no. 2 (1973): 89.

REFERENCES

The following list contains complete citations for works discussed in the Introduction.

Bonica, John J. "Therapeutic Acupuncture in the People's Republic of China." *JAMA* 228 (no. 12, June 17, 1974): 1544–52.

Choain, J. *La "voie rationelle" (Tao) de la medicine chinoise.* Lille: Editions s.l.e.l., 1957.

Dimond, E. G. "Acupuncture Anesthesia, Western Medicine, and Chinese Traditional Medicine." *JAMA* 218 (1971): 1558–63.

Dorf, Paul A. "State Laws Regulating the Practice of Acupuncture." *The Journal of Legal Medicine,* Medical/Legal Aspects of Patient Care. 3 (no. 2, March/April, 1975): 37–40.

Dornette, William H. L. "Acupuncture and the Law." *The Journal of Legal Medicine,* Medical/Legal Aspects of Patient Care. 2 (no. 2, March/April, 1974): 31–38.

Dornette, William Stuart. "The Licensing of the Acupuncture Practitioner—A Legislative Perspective." *The Journal of Legal Medicine,* Medical/Legal Aspects of Patient Care. 2 (no. 2, March/April, 1974): 39–40.

Jenerick, Howard P., ed. *Proceedings N.I.H. Acupuncture Research Conference, February 28, . . . 1973, Bethesda, Maryland.* DHEW Publication no. (NIH) 74–165. Bethesda, Md.: National Institute of General Medicine, U.S. Department of Health, Education, and Welfare, Public Health Service, National Institutes of Health, 1973.

Man, Pang L. and Calvin H. Chen. "Acupuncture 'Anesthesia'—A New Theory and Clinical Study." *Current Therapy Researches* 14 (no. 7, July 1972): 390–94.

References

Mann, Felix. *Acupuncture: The Ancient Chinese Art of Healing.* 2d ed. London: William Heinemann Medical Books, 1971.

———. *The Treatment of Disease by Acupuncture.* London: William Heinemann Medical Books, 1963.

Maspéro, Henri. "Les procédés de 'Nourir le Principe Vital' dans la réligion Taoiste ancienne." *Journal Asiatique* 229 (1937): 177–252, 340–53.

Melzack, R. and P. D. Wall. "Pain Mechanism: A New Theory." *Science* 150 (1965): 971–81.

Morant, Soulié de. Précis de la vraie acuponcture chinoise. Paris, 1935.

Peking Acupunctural Anesthesia Coordinating Group. "The Principle of Acupunctural Anesthesia." *Peking Review* 15 (nos. 7–8, 25 February 1972): 17–18.

Porkert, Manfred. *The Theoretical Foundations of Chinese Medicine, Systems and Correspondences.* Cambridge, Mass., and London: The MIT Press, 1974.

Rasmussen, T. and Wilder Penfield. "Further Studies of the Sensory and Motor Cerebral Cortex of Man." *Proceedings, Federation of Biological Sciences* 6 (1947): 452–60.

Tien, H. C. "Acupuncture Anesthesia: Neurogenic Interference Theory." *World Journal of Psychosynthesis* (1972): 36–41.

Toyama, Philip M. and Michimasa Nishizawa. "The Physiological Basis of Acupuncture Therapy." *North Carolina Medical Journal* 33 (no. 6, May 1972): 425–29.

Veith, Ilza. "Acupuncture Therapy—Past and Present—Verity or Delusion." *JAMA* 180 (May 1962): 478–84.

Veith, Ilza, tr. *Huang Ti Nei Ching Su Wen* [*The Yellow Emperor's Classic of Internal Medicine*]. Berkeley, Calif.: University of California Press, 1966, 1975.

Zulla, H., ed. *Akupunktur in Einzeldarstellungen: Ein Sammel-Doppel-Band mit den Wichtigsten Veröffentlichungen aus 18 Jahrgängen der "Deutschen Zeitschrift für Akupunktur."* 2 vols. Heidelberg: Karl F. Haug Verlag, 1974.

INDEXES

INDEX OF MOST COMMONLY USED ACUPUNCTURE POINTS

Anatomical numbers (*second column, below*). This designation describes the regional anatomical location of the acupuncture point and also identifies the section of the book in which the point is described. The abbreviation

HN designates acupuncture points of the head and neck;
UE designates acupuncture points of the upper extremity;
LE designates acupuncture points of the lower extremity;
CA designates acupuncture points of the chest and abdomen;
B designates acupuncture points of the back.

Thus, HN–1 corresponds to Pê-hui, point #1 in the section "Points of the Head and Neck" in this book.

Meridian numbers (*third column, below*). For the convenience of readers who may be familiar with the so-called Meridian nomenclature for acupuncture points, first popularized in Europe, such numbers are also included in the listing of each point where a comparable Meridian number exists. It should be borne in mind, however, that the Meridian numbering system, dating back nearly one hundred years, has remained static and does not encompass the results of later, and especially the most recent, clinical developments. Consequently, a number of acupuncture points presently used have no corresponding numbers in the Meridian system. The system published here differs slightly from the one in the *American Journal of Chinese Medicine.* In the Meridian system in this book, the abbreviation

Bl refers to the Urinary Bladder meridian;
CS refers to the Circulation-Sex, Pericardium, or Heart-Constrictor meridian;
CV refers to the Conception Vessel or Ren (Front Midline) meridian;
GB refers to the Gallbladder meridian;
GV refers to the Governing Vessel or Du (Back Midline) meridian;
H refers to the Heart meridian;
K refers to the Kidney meridian;
L refers to the Lung meridian;
LI refers to the Large Intestine meridian;
SI refers to the Small Intestine meridian;
Lv refers to the Liver meridian;
S refers to the Stomach meridian;
Sp refers to the Spleen or Spleen-Pancreas meridian;
T refers to the Triple Warmer, Triple Heater, or Sanjiao meridian.

Thus, the Meridian number LI 4 represents point #4 on the Large Intestine meridian, or Ho-ku.

Ch'ang-ch'iang 長強 (anal)	B–25	GV 1	108
Ch'êng-ch'i 承泣 (mid-infraorbital margin)	HN–11	S 1	37
Ch'êng-chiang 承漿 (symphysis menti)	HN–20	CV 24	40
Ch'êng-fu 承扶 (gluteal fold)	LE–3	Bl 36	71
Ch'êng-san 承山 (gastrocnemius)	LE–21	Bl 57	80
Chi-ch'üan 极泉 (axilla)	UE–9	H 1	51
Ch'i-chung 臍中 (umbilicus)	CA–7	CV 8	97
Ch'i-ch'ung 氣冲 (lower inguinal)	CA–13	S 30	99
Ch'i-hai 氣海 (upper hypogastrium)	CA–8	CV 6	97
Ch'i-hai-yü 气海俞 (paravertebral L3–L4)	B–27	Bl 24	108
Ch'i-yin 氣癭 (thyroid)	HN–34	NONE	45
Chia-ch'ê 頰車 (masseter)	HN–9	S 6	37
Chia-ch'êng-chiang 挟承漿 (mental foramen)	HN–21	NONE	40
Chiai-ch'i 解溪 (dorsum, ankle)	LE–13	S 41	76
Chiai-ch'uan 解喘 (paravertebral S1, S2, S3)	B–26	NONE	108
Chiao-kan 交干 (ear point)		NONE	115
Chien-chên 肩貞 (supra posterior axillary fold)	UE–6	SI 9	50
Chien-liao 肩髎 (post-acromion)	UE–4	T 14	49
Chien-nei-lin 肩内陵 (supra anterior axillary fold)	UE–3	NONE	49
Chien-shih 間使 (ventral forearm #2)	UE–25	CS 5	59
Chien-yü 肩髃 (pre-acromion)	UE–2	LI 15	48
Ch'ih-che 尺澤 (antecubital fossa)	UE–20	L 5	57
Chih-kou 支沟 (dorsum, mid-forearm)	UE–14	T 6	54
Chih-pien 秩边 (paravertebral S4–S5)	B–24	Bl 54	107
Chih-shih 志室 (paravertebral L2–L3)	B–16	Bl 52	105
Chih-yin 至陰 (base, fifth toenail)	LE–24	Bl 67	81
Ching-ming 睛明 (medial canthus)	HN–10	Bl 1	37
Ch'iu-hou 球后	HN–12	NONE	38
Ch'iu-hsü 丘墟 (lateral malleolus)	LE–18	GB 40	79
Chiu-wei 鳩尾 (xiphoid process)	CA–5	CV 15	96
Chou-liao 肘髎 (distal humerus)	UE–10	LI 12	52
Ch'ü-ch'ih 曲池 (lateral antecubital fold)	UE–7	LI 11	50

Ch'ü-ch'üan 曲泉 (medial popliteal fold)	LE–31	Lv 8	85
Chü-ku 巨骨 (claviculo-scapular spine angle)	UE–1	LI 16	48
Ch'ü-ku 曲骨 (symphysis pubis)	CA–11	CV 2	98
Chü-liao 居髎 (lateral hip)	LE–2	GB 29	71
Ch'ü-yüan 曲垣 (supraspinous fossa of scapula)	B–8	SI 13	103
Ch'uan-hsi 喘息 (paravertebral C7)	B–3	NONE	101
Chüan-liao, 顴髎 (zygomatic bone)	HN–35	SI 18	45
Chüeh-ku 絶骨 (distal fibula)	LE–17	GB 39	79
Chung-chi 中极 (lower hypogastrium)	CA–10	CV 3	98
Chung-chu 中渚 (inter fourth and fifth metacarpals)	UE–17	T 3	56
Chung-kuan 中脘 (epigastrium)	CA–6	CV 12	97
Chung-tu 中都	LE–40	L 6	89
Êrh-mên 耳門 (superior tragus)	HN–22	T 21	40
Fei-yü 肺俞 (paravertebral T3–T4; lung point)	B–5	Bl 13	103
Fêng-ch'ih 風池	HN–25	GB 20	42
Fêng-lung, 丰隆	LE–41	S 40	89
Fêng-mên 風門 (paravertebral T2–T3)	B–4	Bl 12	101
Fêng-shih 風市 (lateral mid-thigh)	LE–6	GB 31	73
Fu-liu 復溜 (posterior, distal tibia)	LE–35	K 7	87
Fu-t'u 伏兔 (anterior mid-thigh)	LE–5	S 32	72
Fuh-t'u 扶突 (mid-sternocleidomastoideus)	HN–32	LI 18	45
Ho-ku 合谷 (first dorsal interosseous)	UE–12	LI 4	53
Hou-ch'i 后溪 (distal fifth metacarpal)	UE–18	SI 3	56
Hsi-mên 郄門 (ventral forearm #1)	UE–24	CS 4	59
Hsia-kuan 下関 (infratemporal fossa)	HN–8	S 7	37
Hsiao-ch'ang-yü 小腸俞 (paravertebral S1–S2; small intestine point)	B–22	Bl 27	107
Hsien-ku, 陷谷 (inter second and third metatarsals)	LE–42	S 43	89
Hsin-yü 心俞 (paravertebral T5–T6; heart point)	B–6	Bl 15	103
Hsüan-chi 璇玑 (manubrium sterni)	CA–2	CV 21	95
Hsüeh-hai 血海 (medial, supra patella)	LE–25	Sp 10	81
Huan-t'iao 环跳 (posterior hip)	LE–1	GB 30	70
I-fêng 翳風 (post-auricular)	HN–28	T 17	43

I-ming 翳明 (mastoid process)	HN–29	NONE	44
Jen-chung 人中 (Philtrum)	HN–18	GV 26	39
Kan-yü 肝俞 (paravertebral T9–T10; liver point)	B–10	Bl 18	104
Ke-yü 膈俞 (paravertebral T7–T8; diaphragm point)	B–7	Bl 17	103
Kuan-yüan 関元 (mid-hypogastrium)	CA–9	CV 4	97
K'un-lun 昆侖 (posterior, lateral malleolus)	LE–22	Bl 60	80
Kung-sun 公孫 (first metatarsal)	LE–29	Sp 4	83
Kung-tsui, 孔最	UE–36	L 6	65
Lan-wei-hsüeh 闌尾穴 (pretibial #2; appendix point)	LE–11	NONE	76
Lao-kung 勞宮 (distal third metacarpal)	UE–28	CS 8	61
Li-kou 蠡溝 (posterior, mid-tibia)	LE–32	Lv 5	85
Liang-ch'iu 梁丘 (supra lateral patella)	LE–9	S 34	74
Lieh-ch'üeh 列缺 (proximal, styloid process of radius)	UE–21	L 7	58
Lien-ch'üan 廉泉 (supra laryngeal prominence)	HN–33	CV 23	45
Lin-hou 陵后 (posterior, neck of fibula)	LE–39	NONE	88
Ming-mên 命門 (L2–L3)	B–14	GV 4	105
Nao-yü 臑俞 (infra scapular spine)	UE–5	SI 10	49
Nei-kuan 内関 (ventral forearm #3)	UE–26	CS 6	60
Nei-t'ing 内庭 (inter second and third metatarsals)	LE–14	S 44	76
Nei-wai-ch'i-yen 内外膝眼 (para ligament patella)	LE–8	S 35	74
Pa-fêng 八風 (inter metatarso-phalangeal joints)	LE–37	NONE	87
Pa-hsieh 八邪 (inter metacarpo-phalangeal joints)	UE–31	NONE	63
P'ang-k'uang-yü 膀胱俞 (paravertebral S2–S3; bladder point)	B–23	Bl 28	107
Pê-hui 百会 (vertex)	HN–1	GV 20	33
Pi-nao 臂臑 (mid-humerus)	UE–8	LI 14	51
P'i-yü 脾俞 (paravertebral T11–T12; spleen point)	B–12	Bl 20	104
P'ing-ch'uan 平喘 (ear point)	NONE	NONE	115
Ru-kêng 乳根 (nipple line)	CA–4	S 18	95
San-chiao 三焦 (ear point)	NONE	NONE	115

San-yang-lo 三陽絡 UE–35 T 8 65
San-yin-chiao 三陰交 (posterior, distal tibia) LE–27 Sp 6 81
Shang-ch'iu 商丘 (medial malleolus) LE–28 Sp 5 83
Shang-chü-hsü 上巨虛 (pretibial #3) LE–12 S 37 76
Shang-liao 上髎 (first sacral foramen) B–20 Bl 31 106
Shang-pa-fêng 上八風 (inter proximal metatarsals) LE–38 NONE 87
Shang-pa-hsieh 上八邪 (inter distal metacarpals) UE–32 NONE 63
Shao-che 少澤 (fifth fingernail) UE–19 SI 1 57
Shao-hai 少海 (medial antecubital fold) UE–29 H 3 62
Shao-shang 少商 (thumbnail) UE–23 L 11 59
Shên-mên 神門 (medial, ventral wrist) UE–30 H 7 62
Shên-mên 神門 (ear point) NONE NONE 115
Shêng-yü 腎俞 (paravertebral L2–L3; kidney point) B–15 Bl 23 105
Shih-ch'i-ch'ui-hsia 十七椎下 (L5–S1) B–19 NONE 106
Shih-hsüan 十宣 (fingertips) UE–34 NONE 65
Shu-ku 束骨 (fifth metatarsal) LE–23 Bl 65 80
Shuai-ku 率谷 (supratemporal) HN–5 GB 8 35
Szŭ-fêng 四縫 (proximal interphalangeal joints) UE–33 NONE 65
Szŭ-pê 四白 (infraorbital foramen) HN–7 S 2 36
Szŭ-tsu-k'ung 絲竹空 (lateral eyebrow) HN–16 T 23 39
Ta-ch'ang-yü 大腸俞 (paravertebral L4–L5; large intestine point) B–18 Bl 25 106
Ta-ch'ui 大椎 (C7–T1) B–1 GV 14 101
Ta-lin 大陵 (midpoint, ventral wrist) UE–27 CS 7 61
T'ai-ch'i 太溪 (posterior medial malleolus) LE–34 K 3 85
T'ai-ch'ung 太冲 (inter first and second metatarsals) LE–33 Lv 3 85
Tai-mo, 帶脈 (flank) CA–15 GB 26 99
T'ai-yang 太陽 (temporal) HN–3 NONE 34
T'ai-yüan 太淵 (lateral, ventral wrist) UE–22 L 9 59
Tan-chung 膻中 (xiphi-sternal junction) CA–3 CV 17 95
Tan-nang-hsüeh 胆囊穴 (proximal fibula; gallbladder point) LE–16 NONE 79

Point			
Tan-yü 胆俞 (paravertebral T10–T11; gallbladder point)	B–11	Bl 19	104
T'ao-tao 陶道 (T1–T2)	B–2	GV 13	101
Ti-ts'ang 地倉	HN–19	S 4	40
T'ien-ching 天井 (supra olecranon process)	UE–13	T 10	54
T'ien-chu 天柱 (paravertebral C1–C2)	HN–27	Bl 10	42
T'ien-shu 天樞 (paraumbilical)	CA–12	S 25	99
T'ien-tsung 天宗 (infraspinous fossa of scapula)	B–9	SI 11	104
T'ien-t'u 天突 (supra sternal notch)	CA–1	CV 22	95
T'ien-yu 天牖 (post-mastoid process)	HN–31	T 16	44
T'ien-yung 天容 (mandibular angle)	HN–30	SI 17	44
T'ing-hui 听会 (inferior tragus)	HN–24	GB 2	42
T'ing-kung 听宫 (mid-tragus)	HN–23	SI 19	41
Ts'ŭ-liao 次髎 (second sacral foramen)	B–21	Bl 32	107
Tsu-lin-ch'i 足临泣 (inter fourth and fifth metatarsals)	LE–19	GB 41	79
Tsŭ-pao-hsüeh 子包穴 (nose point)	NONE	NONE	228
Tsu-san-li 足三里 (pretibial #1)	LE–10	S 36	74
Tsuan-tsu 攢竹 (superciliary arch)	HN–15	Bl 2	39
T'ung-t'ien 通天	HN–2	Bl 7	34
T'ung-tsŭ-liao 瞳子髎 (lateral canthus)	HN–13	GB 1	38
Tzŭ-kung 子宫 (upper inguinal; uterus point)	CA–14	NONE	99
Wai-kuan 外関 (dorsum, distal forearm)	UE–15	T 5	55
Wei-chung 委中 (popliteal fossa)	LE–20	Bl 40	80
Wei-yü 胃俞 (paravertebral T12–L1; stomach point)	B–13	Bl 21	105
Ya-mên 啞門 (C1–C2)	HN–26	GV 15	42
Yang-ch'i 陽溪 (anatomical snuffbox)	UE–11	LI 5	52
Yang-ch'ih 陽池 (Dorsum, inter third and fourth metacarpals)	UE–16	T 4	55
Yang-lin-ch'üan 陽陵泉 (anterior, neck of fibula)	LE–15	GB 34	78
Yang-pê 陽白 (frontal)	HN–4	GB 14	35
Yao-yang-kuan 腰陽関 (L4–L5)	B–17	GV 3	106

Yin-hsiang 迎香 (nasolabial fold)	HN–17	LI 20	39
Yin-lien 陰廉 (base, femoral triangle)	LE–4	Lv 11	72
Yin-lin-ch'üan 陰陵泉 (posterior, proximal tibia)	LE–26	Sp 9	81
Yin-mên 殷門 (posterior mid-thigh)	LE–7	Bl 37	74
Yin-pê 隐白 (first toenail)	LE–30	Sp 1	83
Yin-t'ang 印堂 (glabella)	HN–6	NONE	36
Yü-yao 魚腰 (mid-eyebrow)	HN–14	NONE	39
Yung-ch'üan 涌泉 (sole of foot)	LE–36	K 1	87

INDEX OF DISEASES AND SYMPTOMS

Amyotrophia 210
Ankle, painful disorders of 215
Appendicitis 207
Asthma 204
Biliary colic 207
Constipation 206
Cough 204
Deafness 212
Dysentery 206
Dyspepsia 205
Elbow, painful disorders of 216
Emesis 205
Enuresis 207
Epilepsy 210
Eye diseases 212
Facial nerve paralysis 209
Finger joints, painful disorders of 217
Gastralgia 205
Goiter 213
Headaches 208

Heel, painful disorders of 215
Hemiplegia 210
Hepatitis 206
Hip, painful disorders of 214
Hypertension 205
Hysterical behavior 211
Ileus (paralytic) 206
Impotence 207
Insomnia 210
Ischemia of extremities 217
Knee, painful disorders of 214
Labor, induction of 212
Lumbago 213
Malaria 203
Mandibular joint, painful disorders of 217
Ménière's disease 213
Menstrual cramps 211
Menstrual irregularities 211
Mutism 212
Nausea 205
Neurasthenia 210
Neurodermatitis 217
Pelvic inflammatory diseases 211
Pharyngitis 204
Poliomyelitis 209
Renal colic 207
Rhinitis 204
Schizophrenia 211
Sciatica 214

Shoulder, painful disorders of 215
Sole of foot, painful disorders of 215
Syncope 203
Tic douloureux 209
Tinnitus 213
Toe, painful disorders of 215
Tonsillitis 204
Toothache 208
Torticollis 217
Upper respiratory infections 203
Urinary tract infections 208
Wrist, painful disorders of 216